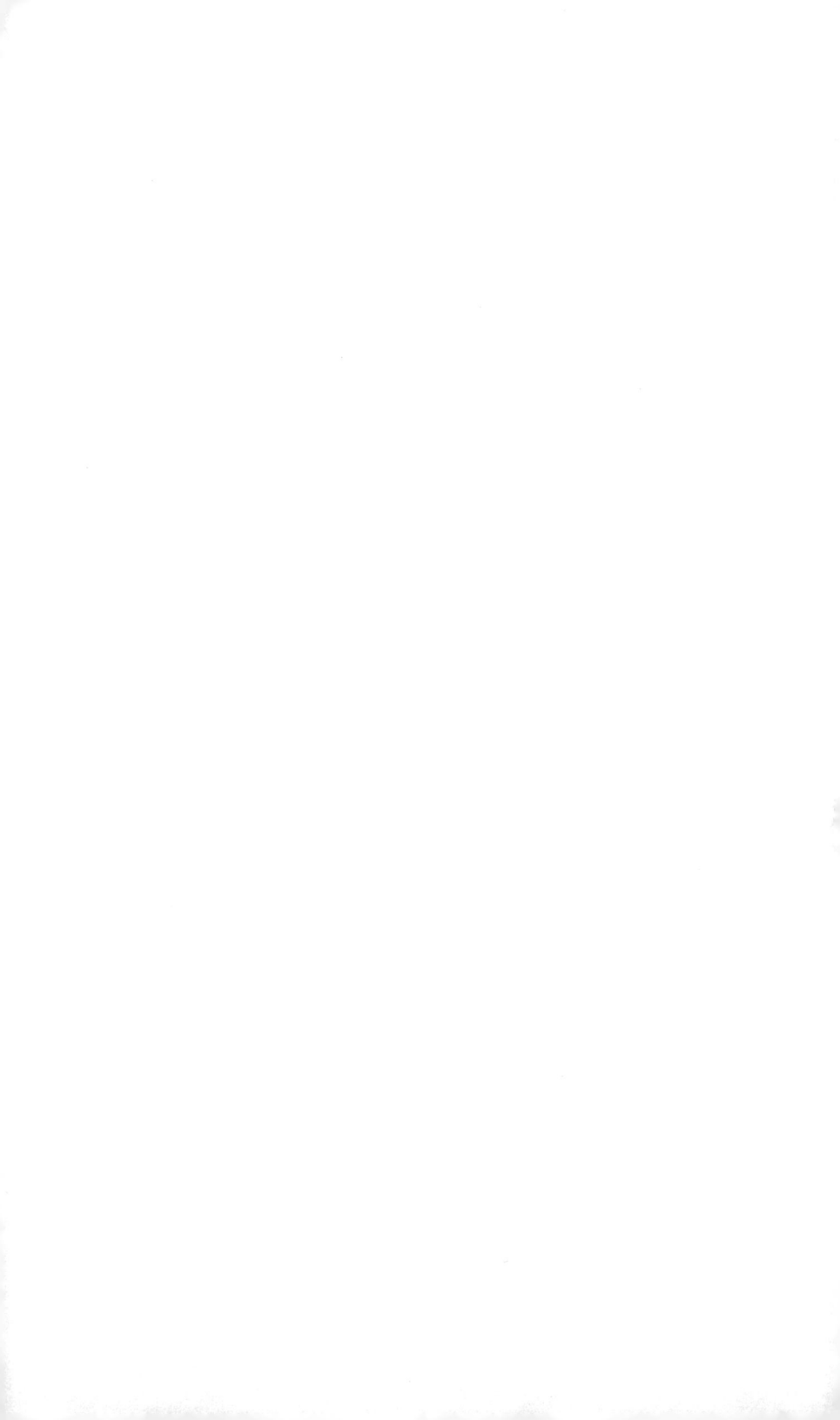

THE MIRACLE OF THE BLACK LEG

Also by Patricia J. Williams

The Alchemy of Race and Rights
The Rooster's Egg
Seeing a Color-Blind Future
Open House
Giving a Damn

THE MIRACLE OF THE BLACK LEG

Notes on Race, Human Bodies,
and the Spirit of the Law

PATRICIA J. WILLIAMS

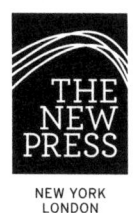

NEW YORK
LONDON

© 2024 by Patricia J. Williams
All rights reserved.
No part of this book may be reproduced, in any form, without written permission from the publisher.

Requests for permission to reproduce selections from this book should be made through our website: https://thenewpress.com/contact.

Published in the United States by The New Press, New York, 2024
Distributed by Two Rivers Distribution

LIBRARY OF CONGRESS CATALOGING-IN-PUBLICATION DATA

Names: Williams, Patricia J., 1951- author.
Title: The miracle of the Black leg : notes on race, human bodies, and the spirit of the law / Patricia J. Williams.
Description: New York : The New Press, 2024. | Includes bibliographical references.
Identifiers: LCCN 2023047985 | ISBN 9781620978160 (hardcover) | ISBN 9781620978238 (ebook)
Subjects: LCSH: Human body--Social aspects--United States. | Human body--Law and legislation--United States. | African Americans--United States--Social conditions. | United States--Ethnic relations. | Race discrimination--United States.
Classification: LCC HM636 .W55 2024 | DDC 306.4/61--dc23/eng/20231027
LC record available at https://lccn.loc.gov/2023047985

The New Press publishes books that promote and enrich public discussion and understanding of the issues vital to our democracy and to a more equitable world. These books are made possible by the enthusiasm of our readers; the support of a committed group of donors, large and small; the collaboration of our many partners in the independent media and the not-for-profit sector; booksellers, who often hand-sell New Press books; librarians; and above all by our authors.

www.thenewpress.com

Book design and composition by Bookbright Media
This book was set in Adobe Garamond and Elza Narrow

Printed in the United States of America

10 9 8 7 6 5 4 3 2 1

Contents

1. Detachment ▪ 1
2. Amputation ▪ 12
3. Lone Ranger ▪ 29
4. Prophylaxis ▪ 44
5. Utopia ▪ 63
6. Making Nice ▪ 71
7. Erasure ▪ 83
8. Process of Elimination ▪ 108
9. Roots ▪ 125
10. Proxy Wars ▪ 139
11. Dogsbody ▪ 166
12. The Dispossessed ▪ 173
13. The Raw and the Half-Cooked ▪ 187
14. Gathering the Ghosts ▪ 200

Acknowledgments ▪ 217
Notes ▪ 219

THE MIRACLE OF THE BLACK LEG

1
Detachment

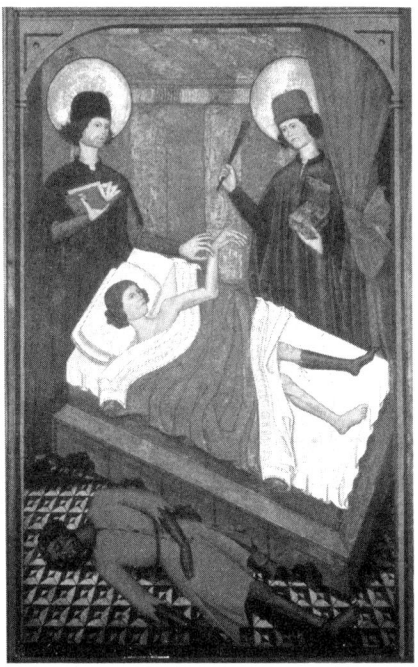

Album/Alamy Stock Photo

I begin this book with a vision of surgery so painful that it has pursued me for several years. It is inspired by an image a student brought me, of the painting above.[1] The student had no knowledge of its provenance, but thought it would intrigue me, given my work with racial representations. It depicts two men with halos—saints? holy men? priests?—presiding over the amputation of a leg apparently removed from an apparently dead Black man. The leg has been attached to the body of an apparently white figure, whom one may surmise is still living, as one of the pontiffs seems to be taking a pulse. It is a religious depiction of some sort, obviously Christian. Having been raised within a loose version of that tradition, I read into its meaning a theology that styles pain as God's chastening, suffering as atonement, agony as God's deliverance.

Still, the lesson of this painting was not clear to me; it was not obvious why the suffering of either the Black or the white man is being sacralized. Furthermore, the composition of the painting is vertically striped with bright red, blood red; to my eye, therefore, there was a river of blood that extends from the top of the frame, grows torrential in the flow of folds of the blanket on the bed, and ultimately coagulates in a pool of red at the bottom, in the cloak of the dead man. Ordinarily I do not flinch at even the most graphic paintings of martyrdom or crucifixion—even John the Baptist's head on a pike. Yet something about this particular picture made my heart batter about with distress. I was surprised to find myself viewing it with such unusual literalism: *it is a centuries-old painting,* my inner originalist and strict constructionist complained; *so this is well before reliable painkillers or anesthesia*! My mind raced with thoughts of the saws and knives that must have been put to the effort. I dreamed of this painting, and I woke up frequently, always worrying that "a leap of faith" was surely a tumble to death with only one leg.

I mulled cluelessly on this painting for almost a year. In my ignorance, my mind composed its own narratives, fillers, titular placeholders, and wandering explanations. The body on the ground was the black sheep, the sacrificial lamb, Epimetheus the Afterthought. The body on the bed was a zombie chimera pieced together from pre-owned bits excavated from a conceptual surplus of others. I imagined that the open book in the hand of the figure in the black cap was an alchemical text containing secrets about some early type of galvanism, or how to transmit electrical sparks of life into used body parts. And I told myself that the open box in the hands of the figure on the right was filled with what surely must be the balm of oblivion.

Upon more recent reflection, I think part of the distress I was feeling was rooted in my vague association with what abolitionist Frederick Douglass wrote in his 1845 autobiography: Douglass famously framed the question of slavery's violence as a kind of amputation. He described his escape from his owner-master in vividly literal economic terms, as stealing the property of his own body, a wrenching theft of "this arm," of "this leg."[2] As "chattel," he was legally disassembled by a system of property in which he had no hand, yet with—and within—which he was intimately, inextricably subsumed. Enslaved bodies were amputated from generative categories like family, citizen, human being. Just as Douglass wrestled with that estrangement, so our body politic lives still with the odd aporia of dark bodies that walk about simultaneously owned, disowned, and fundamentally alien.

Like Douglass, but in the very different context of receiving a heart transplant, philosopher Jean-Luc Nancy was prompted to reflect upon the sense of his body as owned. For Nancy—in contrast to Douglass—it was the *incorporation* of a vital part extracted from another that underwrote his meditation on ownership. He foregrounds his discombobulation that an "alien" heart has taken up residence in his body. Of those moments when his first heart made known its "rebellion, through pauses and arrhythmic lurches," he asks, "If my heart was giving up and going to drop me, to what degree was it an organ of 'mine,' my 'own'?"[3] Nancy even titled his essay "The Intruder" (in his anthology, *Corpus*).[4]

The uncanny force of both Douglass's and Nancy's essays is in part a function of language, of course—the language of property pushed past its normative limits. Both posit unusually painful encounters with notions of possession and autonomy. Both are unsettled by what it means to enunciate "I" and "me" and "mine."

In my own career as a professor of contract law, I teach theories of *Homo economicus*, legal personhood, and the primacy of juridical autonomy. I spend a great deal of time thinking about the body as property, and wondering to what extent any of us are truly "autonomous" rather than just interconnected puzzle bits of each other. Do we have anything like a considered ethic of care for how we borrow, attach, lean on, fit together, or abandon the pieces of one another? Where is it that a single body ends and the complex social webbing of prosthesis begins?

One of the weirder cases exploring this question involved South Carolinian John Wood, whose leg was amputated after an airplane crash in 2004 (and whose subsequent saga is recorded in a sad-funny little film, *Finders Keepers*).[5] Wood, desiring to be eventually buried as a bipedal entity, had the leg embalmed and placed it in a storage unit with other belongings.[6] But he fell behind on the rental fees, and the contents of the unit were sold at auction to one Shannon Whisnant, who found the leg carefully wrapped and nestled inside a barbecue smoker. Whisnant called the police, who traced it back to Wood. Wood insisted the leg be returned, given his sincere belief that, detached or not, it was "his" because it had been part of him. Whisnant, however, asserted that it was "his" because he was what the law recognizes as a "good faith purchaser-for-value." Whisnant hoped to put the leg on display in a homemade House of Horrors, charging a hefty price for the viewing. "Halloween's just around the corner," he explained.[7]

The case of *Wood v. Whisnant* exemplifies how the language habits of rigid contractarianism can contribute to imbalances in the ethics of care and broader public interests.[8] Indeed, the odd icon of John Wood's lost leg is a nearly irresistible subject for allegorizing, uniting it to broader dilemmas of family, market, and language itself—the vehicles of religious communion, community, and cohesion. Thus, it may be legally right but affectively wrong when Shannon Whisnant referred to the leg as his embodied property: "my extra foot." Like any good businessman, he was careful to point out that, by purchasing the smoker and its contents with legal tender, he had thereby incorporated the same into his estate, status, profile, and profit. To top it off, he embraced his *brand* by advertising himself as "the Foot Man."

However, to John Wood the leg was part of "me"—not separable as "a" leg, but rather conceptually indivisible from "himself" or his body. To John Wood, that leg was intrinsically beyond commercial exchange, sacred terrain whose amputation was a symbolic as well as a physical loss. The bony relic was a palpable memorial to the freeze-framed life-changing moment he lost his leg—in the plane crash that killed his father, as well. That leg, removed from the body of which it was formerly an integral part, was a remainder of the day, the marker of a grave.

The ghoulishness of this situation should not obscure the legal issues at stake: should a commodity interest in the contents of the storage unit trump the sacrosanctity of corporeal integrity? Are discarded body parts "alienable" in contract? Or do they fall within the realm of what we deem "inalienable" under the Constitution? The very question foregrounds the peculiar way legal discourses have the power to create wholly incompatible referential worlds. In Anglo-American jurisprudence, contract law concerns itself almost exclusively with the interests of private parties who assign value to the object of their contract according to their own subjective sense of worth. Thus made property, that leg as "object" has no value other than the agreed price of transfer. One definition of property is that it confers a right to exclude. In other words, the value that an owner of an object places upon it excludes or supersedes whatever value it might have had to prior owners or to those not party to the contract. The object is "objectified" precisely because it has no stable or inherent value.

In contrast to contract law, constitutional law governs the realm of polity, civic life, and civil rights. The Declaration of Independence celebrates "Life, Liberty and the pursuit of Happiness" by establishing an *inherency* of civic worth. This is embodied in the notion of legal personhood as "unalienable right"—a human-centered pricelessness that can't be bargained away on an auction block.[9]

Within the meaning-making system of contract law, John Wood's leg becomes an inanimate thing, its status affixed by no one but the storage company and the buyer. Within the semantic realm of constitutional law, however, the leg may be seen as an extension of Wood's dignitarian interest in the integrity of his body, autonomy of mind, and general civic regard. This latter is the ethic that is supposed to protect us, if imperfectly, from the commercial marketing of body parts, and legally shields us from the predations of grave-robbing. This is also the constitutive promise of egalitarian community: that no one of "us" is worth more than another. The core value of constitutional citizenship is that "we" do not eye each other for personal profit, or as prey in extractive mining adventures.

This foundational jurisprudential distinction between constitution and contract—between the vivacity of righted humanity and the civil death of objectification—is at the heart of slavery's complex discursive legacy. While modern concepts of contract have allowed efficiencies of transfer and speculative credit markets to flourish, contract works best when applied to fungible inanimate *things* for which there is an easily determined market price. It works best with inanimate things because the basic remedial scheme for broken contract expectations is usually a narrow one: value promised minus value received. If I paid you ten dollars for magic beans but received only two dollars' worth, you owe me ten minus two, or eight dollars. It does not include punitive damages. It is not designed to deal with the beyond-price-ness of matters such as life and liberty, or pain and suffering, or executions or imprisonment or humanitarian issues.

The 1857 case of *Dred Scott v. Sandford* is an excellent example of the shift in diction from constitutional vivacity to object-of-contract status.[10] Scott had resided in the free territories of Wisconsin and Illinois, and by virtue of his location, he resisted efforts by his "owner" to retain him in the slave state of Missouri as property. Scott, asserting his desired status as a fully agentic human, described John Sandford as "assaulting" him: he used the language of a citizen's claim of criminal and constitutional violation. Sandford, on the other hand, asserted that Scott and his family had been "gently restrained" and returned in good condition: he used the language of bailment, describing Scott like a well-delivered UPS package.

In the same way, Toni Morrison's Nobel Prize–winning novel *Beloved* is based on the real-life case of Margaret Garner, an enslaved woman who escaped from one Archibald Gaines, her rapist and owner, by fleeing from Kentucky across the state line to the free geography of Cincinnati, Ohio.[11] As bounty hunters encircled her, she attempted to kill her young children to spare them a future under Gaines. When her case came to trial in 1856, abolitionists in Ohio, a free state, attempted to have her tried for murder because to do so would affirm her status as an agentic being with the human capacity for willful killing; ironic as it seems, she would thus be better able to assert her status as a free woman and to claim slavery's cruelty as mitigation.[12] Instead, the court ruled her to be chattel—Gaines's "rightful" property, in other words—so under the Fugitive Slave Act of 1850, she was returned to Kentucky as "contraband."[13]

The use of contract to decorporealize human beings via the language of juridical objectification has structural parallels to this day. Consider a world in which there is no governance but the currency of contract: this is, in effect the world described by Jordan Belfort in his hideous memoir *The Wolf of Wall Street*. He describes an office plan to wrap human beings in Velcro suits and throw them at a dartboard to see if they stick; he ponders the trade-off thus: "In essence, what it really boiled down to was that the right to pick up a midget and toss him around was just another currency due any mighty warrior, a spoil of war, so to speak. How else was a man to measure his success if not by playing out every one of his adolescent fantasies, regardless of how bizarre it might be? . . . If precocious success brought about questionable forms of behavior, then the prudent young man should enter each unseemly act into the debit column on his own moral balance sheet and then offset it at some future point with an act of kindness or generosity (a moral credit, so to speak), when he became older and wiser and more sedate."[14] The instrumentalization of fellow humans becomes entirely rationalized by "how much will it cost?" If the price is right, anything goes. It is perhaps more common to frame this critique as one of economics, of neoliberalism writ large. As a student of contract law, I also think of this objectification of human *beings* as the residue of contractarian syntax: a body acted upon, owned by legally assigned agents, one's fate negotiated by disinterested others.

A more starkly politicized example of this instrumentalization came in the summer of 2022, when Florida governor Ron DeSantis played a reductive and dehumanizing referential game by fraudulently luring fifty Venezuelans away from the Texas border, where they had been seeking asylum, and putting them onto a plane that deposited them without notice on the island of Martha's Vineyard.[15] This was done without the consent of and without truthful engagement with the migrants themselves; rather it was a political maneuver to make Democrats in Congress embrace harsher forms of border control. It used migrant bodies as bargaining chips, mere passive tools in a chess game between North and South, liberals and conservatives, sanctuary cities and walled worlds. The migrants' humanity was quite literally "beside the point." Indeed, when the plane sought permission to land on Martha's Vineyard, there was no passenger manifest listing names; according to local rumor, the tower was instead told that the plane was carrying "freight." That the actual human plight of asylum seekers was irrelevant in the political chess of immigration policy became even clearer when, in December 2022, Texas governor Greg Abbott rounded up about 120 people from the border, bused them to Washington, DC, and deposited them on the street in front of vice president Kamala Harris's residence, on the coldest Christmas Eve in the region's history.[16] The temperature hovered at 14 degrees Fahrenheit. The group, including very young children, were abandoned in the road with no winter clothing, some wearing only T-shirts and sandals. Point made, in the transactional game of political tit-for-tat; unlucky human pawns of the game, however, left shivering somewhere far beside that point.

But back to the painting with which I began this chapter. One day I woke up from my spell, finally stopped my clueless imagining about that Black leg stitched onto a white body, and showed the picture to an art historian friend, who unpacked the whole thing for me in under a minute. She informed me that it depicted the Miracle of the Black Leg, as performed by the so-called "Twin Saints, Holy Martyrs, and Silverless (or Unmercenary) Physicians Cosmas and Damian." Cosmas and Damian lived in the third century and are reputed to have performed a series of remarkable healings before they were beheaded by the emperor Diocletian; they are the patron saints of surgery, medicine, pharmacy, and orphaned children.[17]

It turns that hundreds of stories exist about the twin doctors performing that one particular trick of transplantation, more commonly referred to as "The Miracle of the Black Leg."[18] There are many competing stories about the origins of the unmercenary doctors, for Cosmas and Damian are variously tied to the churches of Rome, Asia Minor, and Arabia. The white (or "healed") body is alternately said to be that of Emperor Justinian, or a bishop, or a burgher. And there is much contestation about the source of the leg, the power of that dark appendage pointing to whole different theologies and moral valances: Was it taken from a living or a dead man? An Ethiope or a Moor? A Christian or a Muslim? Was it sacrifice or redemption, resurrection or plucking from the grave? Was the image meant to signify transfiguration from death to life, or was it a mark of some impossibly liminal space, a half and half, the stitching together of like and unlike?—yet still . . . an eternally embodied transgression of one self.

I am glad for the time I allowed my mind to wander loosely over the painting. I pulled odd strands and random associations together as I looked and looked and looked. I invented stories that defied history, time, and place. In the process, I learned a great deal about myself—about the ways in which I prioritized and privileged the pieces of a puzzle for which I had no reasonable process for resolution. For better or worse, I wove myth from the scraps.

For better or worse. My imagination spun cocoons of explanation, like lullabies—once upon a time . . . and thus it shall always be. But as cocooned thoughts will, they sometimes misdirected me with the delights of my own wanderings. Ultimately, I had to step outside of my own assumptions, expectations, and fictionalizing to finally *ask*—thus opening myself to the documentation of the painting's history. I did not have to abandon my own creative musings, but I did have to put them in perspective: to own them as my own, and to set them alongside the larger symbolic universe of this particular religiously inflected symbolic narrative of which I had had no previous knowledge.

In retrospect, I appreciate what had been left out of the frame I had constructed in my own mind. I found alternative meaning for that which was in plain sight but for which I didn't have words. Images are archives, with infinite regressions of reference, of context. Trying to read the narrative of mythic imagery as fluently as the narrative construction of text is always a challenge: figuring out where to delimit the narrative arc—in time, in space, and in the frame. "Documentation" assigns license to see, to envision; it accords creative authority over a story as carried forward. It also presents a basic epistemological problem of how we know the things we know; and of how we become aware of the infinitely complex processes—cognitive, aesthetic cultural, legal—in the production of knowledge.

In a way, my unguided mental wandering implicated the same ethics of completion, accretion, or amendment with which curators, historians, and archaeologists are always confronted: history comes to us in pieces, perpetually unfinished, always in fragmentary form.[19] There is a tension between, on the one hand, trying to understand an unfamiliar text or piece of art by imagining it as a coherent whole to be fixed and formally framed exactly as it once was; and, on the other hand, conceding a lack of certainty and attempting only to identify a pattern, a likelihood, a suggestion. In assembling my own texts, I think of a quote often attributed to Margaret Atwood: "Every utopia . . . faces the same problem: What do you do with the people who don't fit in?"[20]

It is this question, of utopia and its outer rim, that shapes the succeeding chapters of this book—who and what are excluded from our various idealized worlds. I have begun with the example of contract language as existing in some expressive tension with constitutional rights when we talk about human bodies, especially with respect to this country's legacy of the ownership systems of slavery. Throughout, I try to use the lens of the law to explore efforts to preserve those bodies—whole or in part, embryos, severed heads, amputated legs—deemed somehow (and variously) valuable, and to exclude those—via lynching, redlining, selective fertilization, privatization, gun culture, Stop WOKE laws—deemed expendable. Ultimately, this book is my attempt to account for those who don't fit in.

2
Amputation

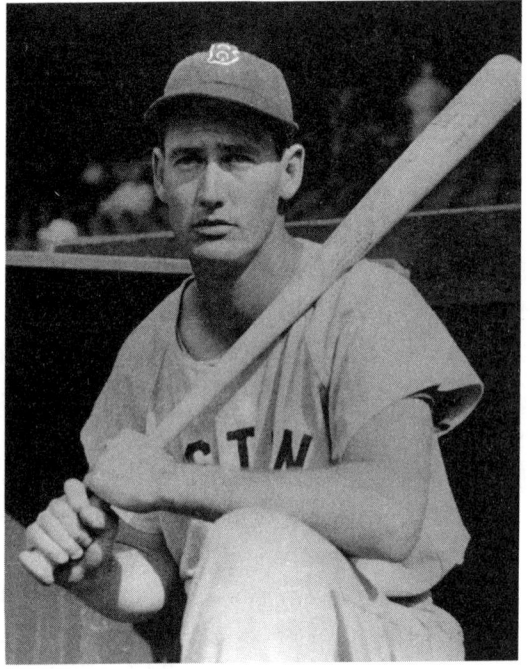

Mark Rucker/Transcendental Graphics/Getty Images

When baseball legend Ted Williams died in 2002, it came to light that he had directed that his body be cryogenically frozen so he and his children would "be able to be together in the future, even if it is only a chance."[1] At the time, it seemed strange to me, a desire for immortality so intense that one would slow the body's decomposition to molecular silence, the breath held in wait for the perfect cure.

What seemed stranger still, however, was the procedure undertaken in pursuit of such putative resurrection: Williams's head was surgically removed from the rest of his body, and the two parts were frozen separately. According to the Associated Press, "The head is stored in a steel can filled with liquid nitrogen. It has been shaved, drilled with holes and accidentally cracked 10 times. Williams' body stands upright in a 9-foot-tall cylindrical steel tank, also filled with liquid nitrogen."[2]

This story makes me sad. When I was a child, Ted Williams was still a living, breathing icon of athleticism. His face was on the packaging of mitts and bats and sports jerseys. He was traded as a baseball card and embodied on bubble gum wrappers. And somehow there was a happily irrational integrity to all that. But while his image always enjoyed a multiplicity of mechanically reproduced lives, his family's stated plan for mechanical disassembly and mechanical *resurrection* resembles nothing more than a badly styled commodity exchange—an econometric form of magical thinking. Cartesian dualism notwithstanding, this elegant and expensive act of butchering was configured as a contract: money paid for the "chance" of immortality. Expressed with a tad less techno-optimism, Williams's children paid $136,000 for two steel vats, a nitrogen-based pickling brew, and what bungled labor it took to perform the "neuroseparation."

Technology may lend us hope, but the language of contract can rationalize even the most absurd acts of hubris. If the question of marketed body parts has always been a focus of philosophical rumination, that conversation has changed in tremendously complex ways in recent years, largely because of revolutionary reproductive, computational, and genetic technologies. Moreover, this particular market—the flesh market, to put it crudely—has ever been susceptible to profane hierarchies of purchased power.

Our era may be what some have called a new industrial revolution—planetary life having been transformed by computers and genomics at least as much as the changes wrought by the steam engine—but cautionary tales about technological hubris have been with us for thousands of years. The demigod Prometheus was punished for his audacity in stealing fire from Olympus and giving it to mortals; angered, Zeus chained him to a rock where an eagle devoured his liver by day. Each night it regenerated, only to be eaten the next day and for all eternity. But Zeus wasn't just angry at Prometheus; he was angry at mortal men for accepting the technological gift of fire. So Zeus sent the first mortal woman, Pandora, down to earth with a little sealed box, a dowry, with instructions that it never be opened. But she was mortal after all, endowed with fallibility and curiosity; she could not resist opening the box, from which the sum of all sins and evils flew out to live in the world—all, except for one small spirit, and that was hope. Hope remained inside.

I think of Pandora when I ponder the ethics of the cryonics company that markets to grieving families a present hope of reversing the putrefaction of death. And I ponder the ethics of families like Ted Williams's, who so incautiously ready themselves to receive the godlike power of life's rekindling. But we are mortal. It's irresistible to grab the torch even when it might burn us badly. We mortals dream of living forever through the grace of all sorts of other technologies than just cryonics. We deploy the magical power of manipulating our future progeny with gene-editing technologies like CRISPR. Some dream of rescuing idealized forms of "pre-born" life by prohibiting contraceptive devices like IUDs or morning-after pills, invoking spiritual concepts of enlivening that would assign molecular independence and full personhood to fertilized eggs from the very instant of conception. Some dream of coding themselves into data bodies that will exceed our biological bodies' life span. Some dream of marrying human minds to seductively chatty extractive computational robots to whose procreations we ought bow down as the authority of "artificial" or "super" intelligence. And some build digital monuments to their lost loved ones, scraping texts, emails, images, and voice messages into whole networked memorial bodies, vivacious gravesites, electronic tombs with avatars that some feel give otherwise deceased bodies a kind of afterlife. There is a combination of yearning and mourning in such thoughts of eternity, self-preservation, or even just self-improvement. And as media anthropologist Brian Michael Murphy writes in his book *We the Dead: Preserving Data at the End of the World*, there is also the risk of hubristic aspirations to a system of technogenesis whereby operationalized "data is circulating through the complex—which includes human bodies and minds—ultimately in service to itself."[3]

Short of full-blown encounters with a dystopian singularity, however, the afterlife of data more often circulates in service to plain old profiteering. Our yearning and mourning and sense of lack is too often fed by monetized technological versions of snake oil. In the general absence of meaningful regulation, American vulnerabilities are assuaged by fabulous fantasies like "medbeds."[4] Medbeds are just plain old beds hooked up to a system that supposedly delivers infusions of "pure biophoton life force energy" unto the worn-down and weary. One such company charges nearly $20,000 for a sealed canister that is labeled a "home generator" of restored health. There is no published explanation or data of what is locked inside the canisters (maybe the ever-elusive Hope, still sheltering in place?), although another company describes the contents as "quantum frequency medicine with scientific proof." Advertisements show images of beds aglow with shimmering circular force fields. What raises a medbed above the ordinary range of consumer fraud, however, is its overlap with the hawking of political fraud as well, and its association with QAnon. According to the BBC, "conspiratorial theorizing includes speculation about 'alien technology' and bizarre claims like the idea that John F. Kennedy, Jr. is still alive, strapped to a medbed."[5]

False advertising and dubious merchant claims don't just dupe the individual consumer who might lose money from a bad bargain. Such practices leach trust from the marketplace and contribute to suspicion and cynicism about other arenas, including public governance and politics. If little can be trusted because hoaxes are more commonplace than rare, then we retreat from civic space with the sense that "nothing is as it seems" and "everyone is out to get us." So much of the world is a fading and dreary old place right now: even I would like to buy the idea that the handsome, cosmopolitan JFK Jr., and his glamorous wife Carolyn Bessette-Kennedy are alive, standing in the wings, hand in hand, waiting to lead us back to Camelot. As a citizen of the most overworked nation on earth, I too want to find purchase in the renewing "life force energy" of eight hours of sleep—in any kind of bed, frankly; but the promise of a little canopy of shimmering biophotons does sound really nice.

The name "medbed," however, suggests medicinal properties, and in the absence of any scientific data showing the same, their sale probably ought to be barred by the Federal Trade Commission as misleading. Vague feel-good promises of curative power are inconsistent with notions of public health and tested science. Unfortunately, consumer oversight agencies have been watered down significantly since the 1980s—since Reaganomics; since the move to shrink all governance, particularly the regulatory structures of the New Deal; and since Ayn Rand's ultra-libertarianism swept American conservatism toward what anti-tax activist Grover Norquist described as a commitment to shrink government so small that it can be drowned in the bathtub. We have returned to many of the laissez-faire policies of the era of robber barons—updated as monopolist techno-kings—and those policies have delivered us to a moment when even the emptiest promises can be styled as freedom of contract, as freedom to trade with whatever fictional or unconscionable value one can imagine, largely unlimited by risk of harm or cautionary principles. The law's already capacious definitions of agency and enterprise become the equivalent of a bored libertarian shrug: "There is no law against stupidity." Or, "It's all on you." If people desperately believe in the capacity to purchase "renewed life" as though it were a commodity . . . well, who's to stop 'em?

My point is that the law of contract should not be the exclusive frame for, well, everything. In Anglo-American jurisprudence, contract is the modern descendant of two ancient English writs: assumpsit and debt. Assumpsit is Latin for "he undertakes" or assumes responsibility to do something. Debt is the writ that imposes payment in exchange for that doing. Together, they join two parties in entirely *voluntary* agreement. As a discursive framework, contract is supposedly enforceable only to the extent that both parties have defined their terms and consented thereto. I speak of this as discursive because the present reality of contract jurisprudence involves little bargaining or haggling, little actual offer or negotiated acceptance. Rather, terms of "adhesion" govern most ordinary contracts today—you're stuck with them. Most consumer transactions are performed online—the little buttons that read "I agree" or "I consent" or "I submit" refer to impossibly lengthy terms that are rarely read—indeed rarely *can* be read by any but the most sophisticated attorney. And even when they can be read and understood, no negotiation is available—there's no "I disagree but would like to proceed anyway" button. Thus, the body of contract has been transformed into more of an automatic trustee relationship beholden to large corporate entities.

Still, in those cases where contract law does involve actual encounter between parties, its structurally reductive power to make property of its objects remains clear and clearly problematic. In the case of *Honeyhline Heidemann v. Jason Heidemann*, a dispute arose between a woman and her ex-husband about the disposition of "cryopreserved human embryos" containing both of their genetic material.[6] The husband argued that it is illegal to treat human embryos as property because they are not appropriate objects of market valuation since they are "unique and not fungible"; and that therefore they are not "goods or chattels."[7] However, Judge Richard E. Gardiner, a Virginia circuit judge, wrote an opinion letter, dated February 8, 2023, concluding that there is no law against buying or selling human embryos; and therefore they should be disposable as personal property. In reaching this conclusion, Gardiner cited the logic of an 1819 Virginia law finding that "all Negro and mulatto slaves shall be held, taken and adjudged to be personal estate." While that law has been updated several times since 1819, Gardiner found that the general language of personal property remains nearly identical today, and hence useful as precedent: "As there is no prohibition on the sale of human embryos, they may be valued and sold, and thus may be considered 'goods or chattels' within the meaning of Code."[8]

Judge Gardiner notwithstanding, trading human beings, or their pieces and parts, through the vehicle of contract is troublesome because modern contract law is a framework largely designed to maximize business interest in "efficient breach" and thus to minimize transaction costs or externalities as much as possible. It is not the easiest vehicle through which to remedy imbalances of bargaining power or accident or negligence or intentional criminality. It is not designed to deal with broad concerns about human need or public accommodation or civil liberties or care for populations in cases of emergency. Other legal structures deal with those eventualities: tort, labor law, criminal law, constitutional law, public health law. Contract should not be the default framework by which we govern ourselves or our polity.

Needless to say, the *Heidemann* opinion has proved a controversial monkey wrench in the ongoing wars about when life begins—even as it surely relies on the ongoing life of slavery's structures.

In September 2014, a white mother named Jennifer Cramblett brought a lawsuit that pursued the question of genetic material as property in unusually literal terms.[9] Cramblett sued an Ohio sperm bank for mistakenly inseminating her with the sperm of an African American donor, "a fact that she said has made it difficult for her and her same-sex partner to raise their now 2-year-old daughter [Payton] in an all-white community," according to the *Chicago Tribune*.[10] Cramblett might have made a claim for negligence in mishandling the vials of sperm with which she was inseminated, for that much is generally recognized in law, having to do with loss of expectation resulting from failure of a duty of care in handling genetic materials. But a different claim is what made Cramblett's case controversial and deeply disturbing: she filed for breach of warranty and emotional and economic loss as a result of "wrongful birth." According to court papers, this claim was explicitly based on the deprivation of whiteness as a trait she thought she was purchasing. Fortunately, the wrongful birth suit was tossed out by DuPage County judge Ronald Sutter a year later, in September 2015. While the story was hot news, the media reflected a rich panoply of social anxieties. Perhaps the most dramatic moment came during an interview with Cramblett on NBC News. "We love her," she said of Payton. "She's made us the people that we are." Cramblett then burst into tears. "But," she continued through clenched teeth, "I'm not going to sit back and let this ever happen to anyone ever again."[11]

That disjunctive, the "but" clause of her despair, was reiterated throughout Cramblett's court papers. Despite being "beautiful," Payton was "obviously mixed-race." While Cramblett purportedly bonded "easily" with the little girl, she "lives each day with fears, anxieties and uncertainty." Her community is "racially intolerant," plus Cramblett suffers from "limited cultural competency relative to African Americans," having never even met one till she got to college. Then there's Cramblett's "all white" family, who can barely stand that she is gay . . . and dear Lord, now this? While Cramblett felt "compelled to repress" her sexual identity among family members, "Payton's differences are irrepressible," the lawsuit states. "Jennifer's stress and anxiety intensify when she envisions Payton entering an all-white school."[12]

Nevertheless, the infant Payton did not make Cramblett and her partner "who we are." They lived a confined and reprehensibly oppressive life before she was born, and it was only because of her birth that they were forced to confront it. The better question is why or how they could have been happy with their lives before.

When Cramblett asserted that her Ohio town was "all-white"—in a state, in a nation, in a world that is absolutely not—one has to wonder how on earth that can be. The sad history of housing segregation in the United States is not a long-ago tale, no matter how much we tend to deny its reality. In 2014, there was a much-publicized encounter between Fox's Bill O'Reilly and Comedy Central's Jon Stewart, during which the two men discussed "white privilege."[13] O'Reilly maintained that his accomplishments had little to do with race and everything to do with hard work. Stewart pointed out that O'Reilly had grown up in Levittown, New York, a planned community on Long Island to which the federal and local governments transferred tremendous mortgage subsidies and other public benefits—while barring Black people from living there—in the post–World War II period. O'Reilly thereby reaped the benefits of a massive, racially exclusive government wealth transfer. As legal scholar Cheryl Harris observed in a 1993 *Harvard Law Review* article, "the law has established and protected an actual property interest in whiteness"—its value dependent on the full faith and credit placed in it, ephemeral but with material consequences.[14]

Bill O'Reilly's Levittown was racially restrictive not only by the developer's private choice; racial segregation was underwritten by federal banking policies and guidelines in the administration of the GI Bill. In the postwar era, not only Levittown but the entire United States became a land divided between "inner cities" and white suburbs because of loan practices that redlined certain neighborhoods if Blacks lived there. Ninety-eight percent of all home loans issued under the GI Bill went to whites, and only 2 percent to people of color. In addition, Levittown imposed a restrictive covenant on homeowners that read: "The tenant agrees not to permit the premises to be used or occupied by any person other than members of the Caucasian race. But the employment and maintenance of other than Caucasian domestic servants shall be permitted."[15]

As Joshua Ruff documents in "Levittown: The Archetype for Suburban Development,"

> In some ways, Levittown resembled the ethnic composition of the military during World War II: Jews, Italians, Irish and Poles living side-by-side. But also like most of the military, African Americans were unable to enter this melting pot. As with many homebuilders in his era, William Levitt didn't question the demands of his financial backers, the FHA, which supported nationwide racial covenants and "redlining"—or devaluing—racially mixed communities. Every Levittown rental lease and homeowner's contract barred those that were "not member(s) of the Caucasian race."[16]

Levitt defended the housing restrictions long after the first residents moved into Levittown, stating that he was just following the social customs of the times. "This is their [the white customers'] attitude, not ours," he once wrote. "As a company our position is simply this: 'We can solve a housing problem, or we can try to solve a racial problem. But we cannot combine the two.'"[17]

Even after the 1948 U.S. Supreme Court decision in *Shelley v. Kraemer* made racial covenants unconstitutional,[18] the FHA continued to underwrite loans only to white neighborhoods. Although Levitt dropped the restrictive language from his leases, he kept up the policy in practice and fought the court's ruling for years afterward. "The elimination of the clause has changed absolutely nothing," he announced in the *Levittown Tribune* in 1949. In 1958, a lawsuit charging discrimination was brought against Levitt in New Jersey, where his third planned community, Willingboro, was being built. In 1960, to avoid public hearings on the case, he agreed to desegregate Willingboro, though the sale of homes to Blacks was highly orchestrated. Racial covenants were not specifically outlawed until the Fair Housing Act, part of the Civil Rights Act of 1968, provided federal enforcement mechanisms.

Long Island's Levittown remains one of the best-documented examples of the long-term distortion that discriminatory mortgage underwriting had in configuring the wealth gap between Blacks and whites. Black people became renters in a land of homeowners because of public policy that denied them access to the same opportunities to accumulate equity in real estate. And for those who were able to afford a home, the very fact of one's skin color lowered its value by virtue of the big redline that would instantly pop up around it. In 2002, one study found Long Island, where Levittown is located, to be the most racially segregated suburb in the entire United States.[19] Things have not budged much since then. While Blacks make up 13.1 percent of America's and nearly 17 percent of New York State's population, as of 2023, Levittown's Black or African American population remains at 1.68 percent.[20]

Jennifer Cramblett exhibited no more awareness of this political history than did Bill O'Reilly. Yet imagine if she and her partner cared about the racism that pervades their environment, instead of suing for the cost of dealing with their "private" distress. Reframed as a civil rights agenda, it might help them to see that they face no more or less than what any Black family faces in the United States.[21] They might begin to consider their claim of individual economic damages more in terms of a civil rights claim for affirmative action and a pushback

Amputation 23

against racial stigma. Perhaps they'd find renewed community and succor by working for fair housing, or by joining Black Lives Matter demonstrations, or by directly engaging with the homophobia and racism among family members as well as in the political landscape.

Instead, Cramblett seemed engulfed by the same race panic that has put the bodies of other children at risk. Little Payton dispossessed her mother by being born, taking the space of a more qualified, more desired white candidate, erupting into the world as damaged goods—a neighborhood defiled as well as a family disappointed. "God's punishment," according to the online hate. "Mistake," according to the court papers. That poisonous geography of mistrust confines us all, whether trapped inside carceral walls at one extreme or gated communities at the other. We are left with a segmented society that does not know itself as whole, our reflection lost in the narrowest shards of a broken mirror.

Let me complicate the picture further: The front page of the March 22, 2007, edition of the *New York Post* offered a fascinating study in the contradictions of our culture.[22]

The top half of the page was consumed by "a stunning mother-child portrait" of Angelina Jolie with little Pax, her newest adopted child, her "Viet man," as the *Post* put it. "See Page Six." The lower half of the page was given over to a lurid headline (BABY BUNGLE: WHITE FOLKS' BLACK CHILD) trumpeting "a Park Avenue fertility clinic's blunder" that "left a family

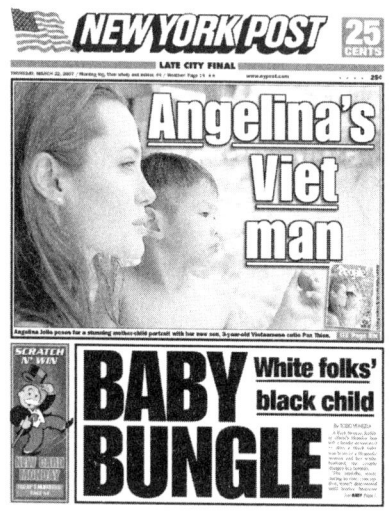

New York Post

devastated—after a Black baby was born to a Hispanic woman and her white husband . . . —"*See* BABY *Page* 6."

I did want more details. I turned to page 6. As it turns out, the *New York Post* has a separate numerical universe in which celebrities romp, whether idolized, idealized, demonized, or drunk. And so the story about Jolie's magical mothering of her rainbow brood was on the trademarked "Page Six"—a gossipy parallel universe of make-believe actually located somewhere around page 14. The bungled baby story, meanwhile, was to be found on "*Page 6*" as determined by the ancient fingers-and-toes methodologies of flat earth. No rainbow magic in this cave: New Yorkers Nancy and Tom Andrews had trouble conceiving after the birth of their first daughter. They employed in vitro fertilization, and baby Jessica was born. Jessica is darker-skinned than either of the Andrewses, a condition that their obstetrician initially called an "abnormality." She'll "lighten up" according to that good doctor. Subsequent paternity tests showed that Nancy Andrews's egg was fertilized by sperm other than that of Tom Andrews. The couple sued the clinic for unspecified damages.[23]

If this were all there were, the story might simply fall within the growing precedent of a number of other technological mix-ups resulting in so-called "wrongful birth" suits for lost eggs, failed vasectomies, botched amniocenteses, etc. However freighted this relatively new area of bioethics may be, there is a general and legally recognized expectation interest that a certain standard of care will be observed in the handling of genetic material, despite the undisputed ethical difficulties with any of these cases, particularly in considering how damages are awarded. Just to start with, it's a bit of a conundrum to call the birth of a healthy child "wrongful." Therefore, courts tend to be conservative in how monetary awards are framed: awarding the costs of raising an unplanned child or one who has health problems resulting from medical malfeasance is obviously less troubling than awarding damages for "the pain and suffering" of parenting a child labeled "unwanted." How does one measure, in dollar or public policy terms, parental "disappointment" at the birth of a baby? Indeed, in the Andrews case, a judge permitted the malpractice claim to go forward but threw out the claim for the mental distress of the parents.

The Andrews case, however, goes a step further than compensation measured by the loss of the father's procreative interest in generation. The Andrewses also (and also unsuccessfully) sought damages for baby Jessica's pain and suffering, apparently for having to live life marooned on an island of Blackness and misery. The judge's opinion quotes the Andrewses concern that Jessica "may be subjected to physical and emotional illness as a result of not being the same race as her parents and siblings." They are "distraught" about what she will do to the family dynamic given that she is "not even the same race, nationality, color . . . as they are." They describe Jessica's conception as a "mishap" so "unimaginable" that they have not told many of their relatives about "the situation." (Telling the tabloids all about it must have come easier?) "We fear that our daughter will be the object of scorn and ridicule by other children, both in school and as she grows up" because Jessica has "characteristics more typical of African or African-American descent." So "while we love Baby Jessica as our own, we are reminded of this terrible mistake each and every time we look at her; it is simply impossible to ignore. . . . We are reminded each and every time we appear in public with her."[24]

There is much to be said about what this construction of affairs will do to Jessica, now old enough to understand; or about the mindset of an attorney who would press a case in such terms; or about why the media could not rein itself in from printing Jessica's real name. But here's the really interesting part. After reading the story in the *Post*, I turned to other media accounts, and it turns out that the *New York Daily News* had embellished the story with a picture of the family—from a 2006 greeting card.[25]

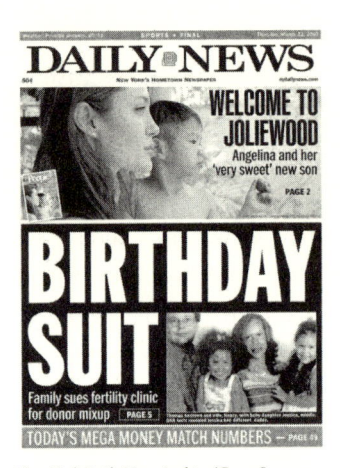

New York Daily News Archive/Getty Images

It is true that Jessica is slightly darker than her mother, and that her hair is somewhat curlier than her sister's, but as one of my students put it, if anything, it is the paleness of the father's skin that marks him as the "different" one.

More than anything else, the picture underscores the embedded cultural oddities of this case, the invisibly shifting notions of how we see boundary, extend intimacy, name "difference." According to the *Post*, Mrs. Andrews is "Hispanic," and apparently one Hispanic woman plus one "white" man equals "a white couple." In other accounts, the mother is "a light-skinned Dominican" which ranking seems to indicate that while she may not be "white," she's surely not "Black." In either event, the narrative seems to imply that if the correct sperm had been used, the Andrewses would have somehow been *guaranteed* a lighter-skinned child. Genetically, though, that's impossible to say, given that most Dominicans trace their heritage to some mixture of African slaves, indigenous islanders, and European settlers, and that darkness of skin color is a dominant trait. Jessica could have been born darker than her mother, in other words, even if Tom Andrews's sperm had been used.

But given a clear mix-up of sperm used for the insemination, one is also left wondering whether the family would have bothered to sue if Jessica had been born lighter than either her mother or sister, or blonder than her father. Regardless of erroneous paternity, would such an outcome have been received as "undesired" enough to provoke such a vehement claim of "wrongful" birth?

These possibilities are entirely absent from the word boxes in which this child is contained. Not only is she viewed as being of a different color than either of her parents, but also of a race apart from either of them and, "even" of a different "nationality"—this latter the most startling for its pure-bloodline configuration of citizenship itself.

Who knows. Maybe my worry is disproportionate. Indeed, I might have consigned all of this to the sensationalized nature of grist for the tabloid mills had I not participated in a lawyerly fracas recently, a strategizing seminar at which this case came up. Well-educated legal minds of all political stripes were arguing that there's nothing wrong in the parents' claim, that it's a private choice they made to have a family that looks "like" them; and why shouldn't they get some money for the girl's "trauma," because after all it is empirically harder to be Black in this society. I could not help noticing that more than a few of the people arguing this stance were the same ones who have argued against affirmative action because we are supposedly such a color-blind society. More significantly, if this reasoning is any kind of reflection of the culture at large, then its logic seems to signal a privatization not merely of family choice, but of the entire Civil Rights Movement. By such calculation, discrimination is no longer a social problem that implicates all of us and our institutions as unloving or less than inclusive. The stigma of difference is positioned as something beyond what we ought to tackle collectively—it's "their choice" after all. Instead, difference becomes destiny, biological defect, eugenic misfortune.

It is filled with irony, this purportedly color-blind time. In an era when none of us is legally defined as a slave but all of us are increasingly objects in the marketplace, it is sad and alarming that "Negro" features, however whimsically perceived or shiftily delineated, still lower the value of the human product, of human grace. It is a cultural perceptual split that scars all of us, even when raised within the most aspirational of families. Matthew Pratt Guterl's memoir *Skinfolk* describes his upbringing in 1970s New Jersey, as the biological son of idealistic white parents who adopted four other children, from Vietnam, Korea, and the South Bronx. Theirs was a deliberate attempt to raise "two of every race" in an "ark for the age of the nuclear bomb, of race riots, of war."[26] But they launched this experiment while living in an otherwise all-white community. The good intentions of his parents notwithstanding, Guterl grew up noting "a troubling public surveillance of our whole ensemble, our various skin tones on display. I watch as cars drive by, and see how quickly the heads turn to see the wide world of rainbow at play in our picket-fenced front yard. A game of catch. A throw of the football. Choosing up teams for Wiffle ball. With Blackness added, our performed comity means something more."[27] Ultimately, the determined intrafamilial discourse of color blindness imposed by his parents led to chasms of silence, disastrous dismissals of traumatic encounters, and outright denials of the differing challenges each child faced in an often-intolerant world. "As children in a family meant to undo racism, we were asked to learn—and to unlearn—race. To see one another as siblings—to see beyond our skin—but also, dissonantly, to see one another as color-coded. . . . Those parallel lessons are, in the end, impossible to suture together."[28]

This, after all, is a feature of American life succinctly captured in that split front page of the *New York Post*: the troubling cultural doublespeak of neo-/bi-/post-/inter-racialist confusions—-the Vietnamese-born Pax and the Cambodian-born Maddox and the Ethiopian-born Zahara all enjoying the ethereally perfumed embrace of Angelina Jolie, versus the local, on-the-ground "disaster" of being born Jessica.

3
Lone Ranger

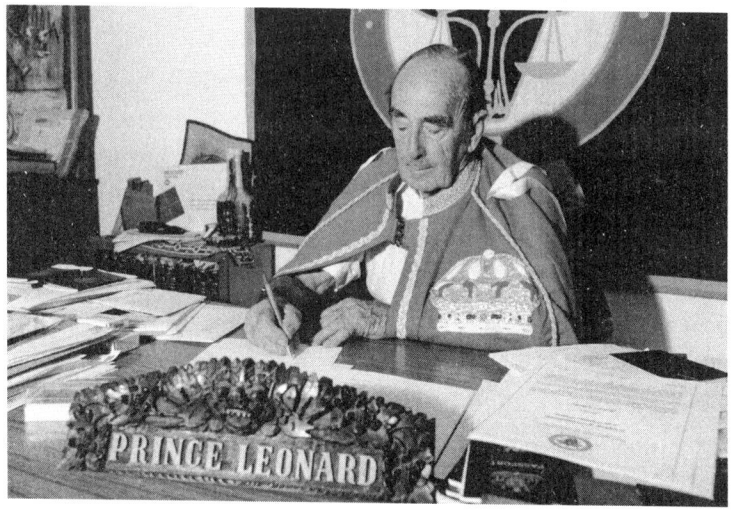

Hemis/Alamy Stock Photo

From 1970 until August 2020, an eccentric Australian wheat farmer named Leonard Casley set himself up as the royal figurehead of what he dubbed the Principality of Hutt River. In a fit of pique growing out of a dispute over wheat tariffs, he declared that he and his eighteen-thousand-acre property were seceding from Australia to become an independent nation state, with the power to fly its own flag, to run its own post office, to issue its own passports, visas, and currency, and to raise its own army.[1] The whole enterprise became a kind of long-standing joke—as well as a thriving tourist attraction—with the Australian government making only half-hearted efforts to collect its long-overdue taxes (at least until Prince Leonard's recent death, when Australia swooped in to force payment from sale of some of the land).[2]

I raise that strange little story here because it is a gentler, funnier version of the more ardent cowboy or "frontier" individualism that seems to have reemerged with such force here in the United States. Within this ideological zeitgeist, every man—for it so often seems to be a man—is waging his own personal civil war, declaring sovereignty, declaring independence from all governmentalism. It's a way of thinking about liberty that does not easily comport with public accommodation and equality notions under civil rights laws. Rather, it asserts a right to be altogether lawless, or to make one's own law. In effect, it advances a purported right not merely to "stand your ground" in the context of self-defense, but an individual right to put a standing army on ground that you have claimed merely by virtue of your standing on it. As with actual stand-your-ground laws, the flaw in this is the degree to which any given princeling's subjective feeling about what's a lethal threat privileges the last one standing after shooting first and asking questions later.

As performative practice, the Sovereign Man is everywhere, from Jeff Bezos colonizing space in cowboy regalia to Lil Nas X's parody of the same.

The endless body-posturing, the G.I. Joe militarized cosplaying, the standing up, the standing back, the standing down—this brand of libertarianism depends on collective norms despite itself: it is enmeshed in sloshy affective power relations having to do with race, phenotype, class, gun culture, caste, and interpersonal context. It is an unfortunate truism that white men flexing their muscles with military-grade weapons in demonstrations against state legislatures or local school boards are tolerated to very different degree than would be similar posses of Black men armed to the gills. Moreover, the "open carry" of long arms and machine guns has a longer shadow related to

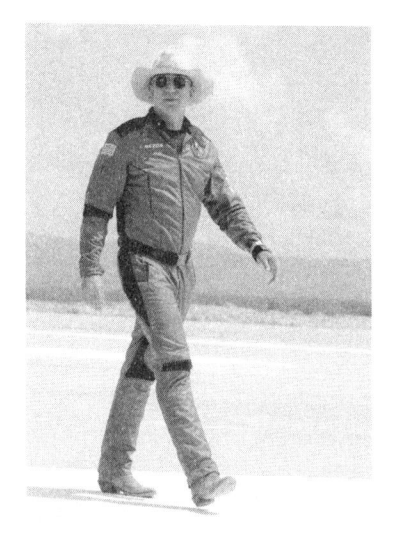

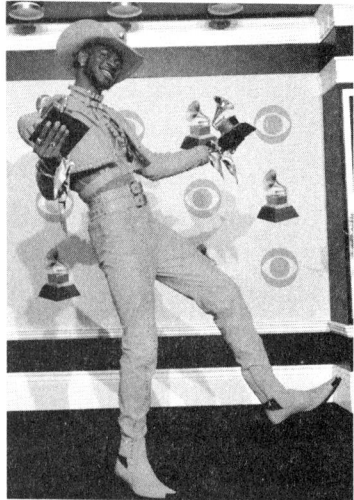

Joe Raedle/Getty Images   Alberto E. Rodriguez/Getty Images

the distributed power of vigilantism, licensing private actors, largely in the South, to "hunt" fugitives for bounty, a practice that is nearly identical in its framing to the Fugitive Slave Act.

The Fugitive Slave Act gave reimbursement power to local authorities when slave-catching required them to "summon and call to their aid the bystanders, or posse comitatus of the proper county . . . and all good citizens are hereby commanded to aid and assist in the prompt and efficient execution of this law."[3] In similar fashion, Florida's "Stop WOKE Act" does not just ban "uncomfortable" books.[4] It de-professionalizes teaching by distributing enforcement power to a disunited plethora of parents: The law gives parents the power to sue school districts if they teach anything related to gay or trans existence, or if they teach anything about what remains undefined but vaguely designated as "critical race theory." It allows parents to collect monetary reimbursements and attorney fees. And Texas's antiabortion law, SB8, not only criminalizes abortion; it deputizes private citizens for its enforcement, allowing any individual to sue in civil court any other person who "aids or abets" an abortion.[5] The law's promise of civil awards up to $10,000 for such suits provides financial incentives for outsourced policing and citizen arrest.[6]

Pending lawsuits are lining up to challenge such bounty schemes, but from *Dog the Bounty Hunter* to the Oath Keepers, there is a resurgent trend to concede governance to a welter of what are effectively privatized standing armies. An incoherent patchwork of individual civil wars and small revolutions is declared daily against school boards, voting machines, the National Institutes of Health, the humanities, gun control, and just thinking before opening one's mouth. All this operates to destabilize the professionalism of trained law enforcement, trained teachers, trained doctors and nurses, trained scientists, trained diplomats. The massive and unprecedented implosion of faith in tried-and-true best practices—in everything from education to medicine to political codes of conduct—endangers us all.

That power of unapologetic ultra-singularity is a very particular kind of privilege: being no-more-than-one means that one's actions do not signify for all others "like you" because you are "naturally" defined as a lone wolf, naturally unique, naturally autonomous. It follows, naturally then, that the sovereign makes his own rules; naturally, all who enter his territory do so at the sovereign's pleasure. The very figuration of going solo invokes an imaginary landscape where multiple plural others exist only to be kept behind the wall, beyond the moat, outside the pale. In that landscape, those marked as "other" must survive the unprivileged precarity of being perceived as the object of, and being objectified by, the worst fears of randomly encountered strangers.

There is much to fear in our well-armed culture, at this technologically electrified moment. Those marked as others or strangers can shift in an instant—with a tweet or an Instagram story. The focus bounces around like a kitten in Kevlar chasing a laser beam. One moment it's "liberal governors" like Ralph Northam or Gretchen Whitmer; then blood-sucking pedophiles in nonexistent pizza-shop basements; then Dr. Fauci; then Nancy Pelosi; then Nancy Pelosi's husband's invisible (and entirely imaginary) gay lover.[7] Never have unsubstantiated fears been given such militarized weight. It's as though Americans have PTSD, responding to the slightest rustle as though it were an explosion. Perhaps indeed we are all traumatized beyond capacity for common sense.

Meanwhile, as a general longer-term matter, there is both paradox and pattern: the conceptually "lone" sovereign citizen often makes war against stereotyped bodies rather than real enemies. In present-day America, those most statistically likely to be objectified as unbridled "theys" or "thems" are women, people of color, religious minorities including Jews and Muslims, and immigrants. The "they" marks a body as plurally iconic; such a "them" replicates darkly, signifying unknown risks, exploding with excess armies of meaning.... It is no wonder that the stably singular lone-wolf citizen soldier, that the brave army of one, might think he needs a rocket launcher.

Ironically, to be any kind of "them" is to be the target of a plurality of singular sovereigns: millions of self-declared potentates or self-appointed security guards (à la George Zimmerman); people who daily impose thousands of self-proclaimed checkpoints for "thems," each threshold ruled by a different subjectivity of rules and whims and deadly fears. That power of demarcation is always shifting, indeed the entire world becomes "shifty." It is epitomized by the sad phenomenon of some sovereign citizens and militia members mustering to protect homes and businesses during the worst of California's forest fires, inspired to do so because of baseless internet rumors of supposed "antifa" arsonists and looters. Despite official police and professional fire departments begging them not to rush in and create more confusion, some eager sovereign citizens self-deputized and ended up chasing themselves, mistaking one another for the enemy, as they ran through the reality of a ravaged and densely smoky landscape—as they ran at the same time through the simulated reality of their own imagined hellscape.[8]

This radical form of individualism makes community space a dystopia of individual principalities, each its own tense little war zone, its own guarded turf, apt to erupt without warning. These projections of freedom as ultimate control are accompanied by a form of subjectivity fantasized as immune to consequence—sovereignly immune—because these personal fiefdoms are defined as *inherently ungovernable*. This extreme form of libertarianism rationalizes itself, the one-and-only-self, as resolutely singular even when staring down webs of life in which we are all invisibly and irretrievably enmeshed—both institutionally and biologically. And it undermines anything like federalism or unity of states.

This collection of uncollectibles is governed differently. Power from the top is almost gaseous: suggested but not coordinated, envisioned but not encoded, insinuated but rarely stated. As a result, no single person or institution can easily be brought to account.

Furthermore, matters that used to be the province of constitutional discourse have been downsized and outsourced and pushed into the realm and the discourse of private contract. Private schooling, private prisons, pay-to-play for what used to be thought of as public goods, public utilities, public spaces, including fire departments and parks. That kind of arch-transactionalism changes the nature of both the thing being exchanged in contract as well as the "we" who are supposedly constitutionally autonomous agents.

Remember, again, the way that John Wood's leg changes its nature when it's governed not by the norms of private contract but by constitutional discourse. It shifts from being a commodified thing to a relic of his humanity, an extension of regard we might call spiritual. Constitutional rights create a dignitarian space that we provide to one another: a sphere of control over the body that we do not violate as a matter of constitutional value. This is not the same as contract's limited metric of cost-benefit value. Instead, the leg is positioned as beyond ordinary price, non-fungible, neither goods nor chattel.

John Wood's claim about the leg, like Jason Heidemann's claim about the frozen embryos, demonstrates the existential question at the heart of legal differentiations between those interests that pertain to our humanity and collective flourishing, and those interests that pertain to fungible, tradeable, insensate objects of property. This deliberation is most vexed when human bodies, pieces of bodies, or interests in bodies enter the marketplace: labor, prostitution, grave-robbing for profit, surrogacy contracts, some nonmedical cosmetic surgeries, gene editing that makes a product of "designer babies," etc. Sale of bodies or their parts usually involves some form of detachment, or a compromise to what we think of as integrity of the body and its autonomy. It may invoke therefore problems of dignity or civic respect, depending on the intimacy of what is detached—physically or conceptually. Selling one's shorn hair as a marketable thing is less concerning than selling something non-fungible—that is, not easily replaceable—like one's kidney, for example.

Some will recall the story of Wang Shangkun, a broke Chinese seventeen-year-old who sold his kidney in 2011 in order to purchase an iPad and an iPhone4. "Why do I need a second kidney? One is enough," he was quoted as stating rather brashly.[9] But the reason such marketized transactions are universally illegal is that vital organs are precisely that: vital—non-fungible, irreplacable, beyond ordinary price. And so the doctors who performed his operation were arrested and charged with organ trading on the black market. Shortly thereafter, moreover, the unfortunate Mr. Shangkun suffered severe postoperative infections and renal failure. He will require dialysis for the rest of his life . . . unless, ironically, he can find someone to donate a kidney to him.[10]

Years ago, at the height of what in the Western world was known as "women's lib," I remember a defector from the Iron Curtain scoffing at the Soviet Union's claim that it had achieved complete sexual equality: "When a woman advances in the factory, it's only after they hold a beauty contest." Perhaps the story was apocryphal, but it made me think about Ralph Ellison's great novel *Invisible Man*, in which the Black narrator is awarded a college scholarship for his oratorical skills. When he presents himself to receive the award, however, he is first required to strip and to engage in a boxing match styled as a "battle royal," and then to scamper across an electrified rug chasing tossed gold-foil tokens. When he is finally presented with the scholarship scroll, he reflects on what has turned out to be the trade of his dignity and imagines that it really reads "To Whom It May Concern, Keep This Nigger-Boy Running."

The brute survival economy of booty or boxing competitions also makes me think about rapper Juicy J's offer some years ago of a $50,000 college scholarship to "the best chick that can twerk." Despite Mr. J's lasciviously descriptive flair, it struck me as not all that different from Miss Universe contestants parading their bikinied bodies in hopes of a similar prize. (Which is more unsettling, having the exchange rate of one's assets fixed by Juicy J or by Donald Trump?)

I cite these examples not to debate the propriety of selling one's body—an open question—but to consider its perceived necessity. Amid a squeezed labor market and stratospherically rising tuition costs, new flesh markets are burgeoning among the middle class, particularly upwardly aspiring young women. I have written before about how many of my students have "donated" their "Ivy League" eggs to wealthy women who pay upward of $50,000 per "harvest" if they can meet certain metrics of height, weight, eye color, athleticism, and SAT scores.[11] Egg extraction is risky and invasive, but it is, I am told, an easier way of putting oneself through school than a job at McDonald's.

By the same token, consider a poll by Seeking.com (formerly SeekingArrangement.com) which pairs older, wealthy men and young women—"sugar babies"—for "mutually beneficial relationships."[12]

The site has claimed that the average sugar baby receives $3,000 a month and that 44 percent of its U.S. clientele are college students, a significant minority of them single mothers. Of nine hundred female students at Arizona State University polled, 68 percent said they would use such a service.[13] Indeed, one YouTube video showed a procession of students holding signs reading I Need a Sugar Daddy for . . . The litany of needs included books, tuition, and law school. Some were seeking more frivolous things, like designer clothes or "boobs," but despite their giggly demeanor, to me they recalled the images of cardboard placards in Depression-era Hoovervilles reading Will Work for Food.[14]

While such "luxury" dating sites deny that they are engaged in pimping, there's a wink-wink element to the coy policy of leaving it up to each couple to define what is being sponsored. Sex is never mentioned, but it's hard to make a clear distinction between the playful come-hither posture of the young women and the overly practiced smiles of prostitutes in the windows of any given red-light district.

When such sites were still a relatively new phenomenon, Dr. Phil hosted a panel of sugar babies who described themselves as free agents, whose "arrangements" did not "necessarily" involve sex, and who said that sex work is something that happens on street corners.[15] My goal here is not to decide whether this is a wholesome expression of sexual freedom or a new low in prostration before the dollar. But even if upheld as a purely "rational economic choice," I wonder if most women wouldn't honestly prefer to get their education or earn their livelihood without having to satisfy the "companionship" whims of strangers. In this sense, the dilemma is not just about prostitution or mutually assumed contracts, but also about the marketed nature of a range of exchanges—even marriage—that are broadly gendered, classed, and raced (particularly if we include those who actually do work on street corners).

The story of former model Sara Ziff, founder of the Model Alliance, is instructive. Recruited by a top agency when she was fourteen, she has described the dark side of a job that most people imagine as glamorous: long hours, sexual exploitation, being treated like a piece of meat.[16] Ziff's activism centers partly on the fact that models earn, on average, just $27,000 a year, but she's at her fiercest when it comes to the indignities for which no sum of money is enough: the encounters with men in the business whose harassment, or worse, makes you want to jump out of your skin.[17] Ziff worries about the ways the degradation that models experience is cloaked in discourse about free choice, rationalized as fair—even lucky. After all, isn't it ingratitude to gripe about exploitation if a woman has sufficient "hotness" to sell (as one young woman described it to Dr. Phil)?

Back in the 1970s, Marabel Morgan published her evangelical marriage manual, *The Total Woman*. It advocated the complete submission of wives to their husbands, with tips for ensuring that he won't leave you destitute. (Greeting your hubby at the door with a tray of martinis while dressed only in Saran Wrap was one of her more famous ideas.) That women still often look to men to lift them out of destitution is part of a larger American picture: as of 2022, it costs over $310,000 to raise a child to eighteen;[18] federal and state subsidies to colleges and universities have been compromised or slashed as tuition steadily rises.[19]

We could simply shrug all this off and conclude that "Self-Exploitation 101" is the chief skill set to fall back on as the wealth gap grows and the social safety net is shredded. But what of the educational, moral, and citizenship costs in a world of invisible women—and not a few invisible minorities, immigrants, and indigents—flashing their bodies and leaping at the scrip tossed out at the private clubs of wealthier, mostly male plutocrats?

Those costs to citizenship perhaps become clearer when participatory democracy itself is put on the auction block, with civil rights traded off as privatized choice. Senator Rand Paul of Kentucky (whose father, former senator Ron Paul, named him after individual-egoist Ayn Rand), illustrated such a trade-off when he stated his belief that the Fair Housing Act is wrong because "free society will abide unofficial, private discrimination, even when that means allowing hate-filled groups to exclude people based on the color of their skin."[20] Similarly, John Cook, member of the Texas State Republican Executive Committee, expressed his desire to privatize even a public body like the Texas House of Representatives by suggesting that Republican Joe Straus, who is Jewish, be replaced as speaker of the Texas House of Representatives because "we elected a House with Christian, conservative values. We now want a true Christian conservative running it."[21] And Judson Phillips, founder of the Tea Party Nation, has endorsed "the original intent" of restricting voting rights to citizens who are property holders because "if you're a property owner, you actually have a vested stake in the community."[22] Policies originally promulgated to maintain economic supremacy by controlling the movement, political status, and access to property of Blacks, Jews, and poor whites in the Deep South seem to have come full circle.

One vivid trace of these policies of control can be seen in the fate of Gene Cranick, an elderly, wheelchair-bound white resident of Obion County, Tennessee. When a backyard trash fire spread to his house in October of 2010, he called the fire department. The firemen came, parked in front, but leaned against their trucks and watched Cranick's property—and the animals within the farmhouse—burn to the ground.[23] Yet they hosed down the neighbors' houses on either side. Why? Because Gene Cranick's house was in an unincorporated part of the county, beyond the city limits, where a so-called "pay-to-spray" system was in place. In that area you had to choose to buy into the fire department or not. It's an "opt-in" system, a system of free choice, individual preference. You pay $75 a year and you get fire department service. If you don't pay, you get nothing. Cranick's neighbors had paid the $75. Cranick had forgotten to pay that year. The fire department took care of the neighbor who had paid. And when the fire on Cranick's property spread to another field belonging to a third neighbor who hadn't paid, the fire department watched that land burn as well.[24]

Cranick offered to pay the actual cost of putting it out, but the fire chief operated according to the logic of Cranick's being a "free rider"—and refused to service him because to do so would incentivize others to make bad economic choices.[25] Moral hazard trumped material hazard. And so the fire department let the fire have its way, racing to ungovernability, evidently uncontrollable by private contract. Fire, after all, is a force that operates according to its own dynamic; it is not contained by individual selection and private preferences.

In the wake of publicity about this case, media analysts weighed in. On MSNBC, liberal commentator Keith Olbermann decried the lack of a public spirit and the dearth of an ethic of res publica.[26] Conservative radio host Glenn Beck and the *National Review*, by contrast, engaged in heated defenses of pay-to-spray systems, invoking Pareto optimality and complex analyses of the free-rider problem.[27] Glenn Beck derided those who sympathized with Gene Cranick in very succinct terms: "Compassion, compassion, compassion! It's not about compassion! It's about the $75!"[28] The competing narratives offered a fascinating study of comparative discourses: in the narrow market logics of contract-speak, fire was configured as bounded, a consequence that could be contained to the decision-making rationalities of a single actor. Payment was located as the central moral value. But from a constitutionally civic-minded frame, fire is treated as a shared threat, a public harm, whose potential for ignoring human boundaries poses risks, against which we pool our resources for the collective good. Public health and safety become the central moral values.

Note, too, the way Gene Cranick's status shifts depending on where he's located in this geography. If you wonder why any town or municipality or government structure would treat fire in this way, it's because opt-in systems are almost exclusively located in geographies reserved for people who were not historically treated as full citizens, or where the monetary cost of extending public services is deemed to exceed the human value or social interest. It is the manifestation of a moral hierarchy: that which is located in the realm of extreme privacy and individual control is treated as that which is of no interest to others. The fate of those existing in that tight little zone is "no one else's business." It is a closed kingdom of personal preference. Paradoxically, such a configuration may be a great boon to corporations or to gated communities or to those who are independently wealthy—i.e., those creatures who flourish in closed terrariums, and need no help to survive in our complexly interconnected world. But if private choice is applied as the exclusive metric of moral governance, then such an explicitly antisocial stance falls hard upon those who must rely more heavily on public utilities, shared resources, and communally governed infrastructure, including road and sewer maintenance, garbage pickup, electrical grids, libraries, schools, and communications infrastructures.

Gene Cranick was white, but I think of him as an actuarial Black man, because he had the misfortune to live in an unincorporated area that had the limited services historically associated with Black neighborhoods. Under Jim Crow, publicly shared amenities such as fire, sewer, and police services would often stop at the edge of a town based on the lines of segregation. For example, historian Richard Kluger's book *Simple Justice* relates how civil rights activist Joseph DeLaine's South Carolina home was apparently targeted by arsonists in the 1950s: members of the all-white Summerton fire department were on hand as the wooden house burned to the ground, but they made no effort to put out the flames because DeLaine's house, they said, was beyond the town limits. And it was: by one hundred feet.[29]

This form of racialized exclusion from public utilities scars the geographies of Black neighborhoods to this day, particularly in the

U.S. South, in former slave states. These systems mark the landscape of prejudice, where public protection stopped and private individualized payments have had to stand in. Residents must opt in for all sorts of privileges, individual by individual, a paradoxical kind of ticket onto the freedom train. These demographic patterns can be overlaid almost precisely upon the cartographic inscriptions of plantation arrangements. Hence, opt-in fire departments don't exist in many places outside the South; those raised in places where civic destiny is conceptually shared may find the idea of a "private" outbreak of fire utterly incomprehensible.

In contractualized thought systems like this, invisible histories continue to play out under the radar. They may express themselves as purely budgetary choices, but they recapitulate what living "beyond the pale" has meant in other geographies of historical deprivation, like England's rule of Ireland, or Imperial Russia's imposition of the Pale of Settlement. Many of our most pronounced racial disparities in American life bear the quiet footprint of intergenerational habits of thought about whose lives matter and whose don't, who belongs and who does not, who can pay and who can't play.

For example, de facto segregation in public schools is frequently enforced by ostensibly "race-neutral" laws against "boundary-hopping" across school districts, swaddled in the innocent language of "my" tax dollars as opposed to "yours." One of the saddest consequences of America's uniquely local tax-based school funding system is exemplified by those cases where poor, almost always Black parents are sued or jailed for lying about their addresses so they can send their children to well-resourced schools in better (almost always whiter) neighborhoods. The charge is called "theft of education."

Think of the case of Kelley Williams-Bolar, who used her father's address in a nearby suburb to move her children from a dilapidated school in the city of Akron that met only four of Ohio's educational standards to one that met and exceeded all twenty-six of the state's guidelines. The school hired investigators to follow her around and found that the children were living with their grandfather only five days a week, returning to their mother on weekends. In 2011, Williams-Bolar and her father were charged with felonies: falsification of records and theft of public education. She was given two five-year jail terms, suspended; she ended up serving nine days in jail, plus three years of probation and eighty hours of community service.[30]

The same unfortunate logic underwrote the catastrophe befalling Flint, Michigan, where the entire population (more than half of whom are Black) was poisoned by prolonged exposure to high levels of lead. The diversion of Flint's public water system was imposed on it by a governor interested only in "cost-cutting." Oversight of the new system was then outsourced and made lean in a way that evaded public accountability and resisted massive public protest about the water being putrid and contaminated. Governor Rick Snyder's promise to his largely Republican constituency was that all government be run "like a business" and that slashing services somehow amounted to public profit. Cutting costs led to cutting corners. As a result, Flint's entire population endured prolonged exposure to high levels of lead poisoning, and a generation of children was permanently developmentally damaged.[31] But while health of the residents plummeted, money was saved, ledgers were balanced, and budgets with no fat were touted like proud anorexics on Instagram.

As Glenn Beck said of Gene Cranick's losses, "It's about the $75!"

4
Prophylaxis

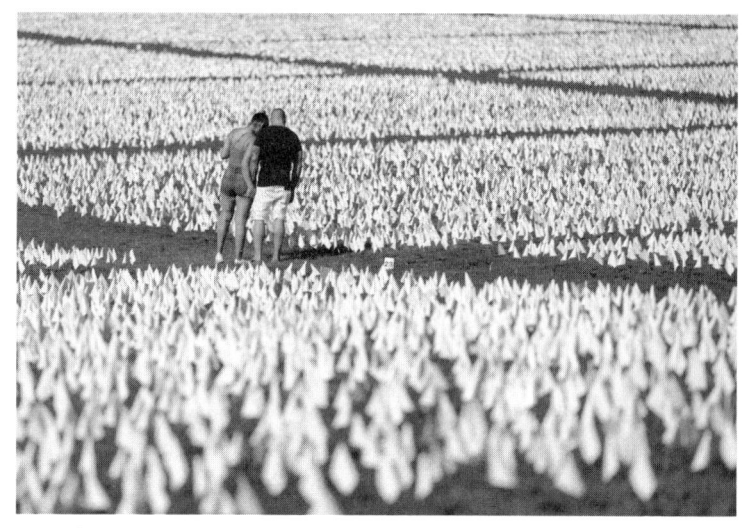

Kent Nishimura/*Los Angeles Times*/Getty Images

In mid-March 2020, the COVID-19 pandemic exploded globally and exponentially, upending the world.[1] Friends began to die, the social gave way to the solitary; both moral panic and contagious disease "spread like wildfire."[2]

As the case of Gene Cranick's house fire might suggest, mass catastrophe may not be the most effective field of operation for theories of individual choice. "Help, help!" seems a more usefully collaborative directive: a call for collective response, a call for the bucket brigade, a call for "all hands on deck" to pitch in. "Help!" was certainly what I prayed for in early 2020 as ambulance sirens wailed all day and into the night. Indeed, the immersive panic that gripped the world in those early days of COVID's voracious spread initially made me hope against hope that the enormity of the plague would equalize us in our felt susceptibility. All people, as living organisms, are vulnerable to the predations of this disease, so I did not question what seemed to me the obvious need for all powers to wave a white flag and set aside lesser issues. We would fight this conflagration with determined unity, I thought, and band together in a florescence of knowledge sharing so that our species might survive.

I am among the first generation who profited from microbiologist Jonas Salk's formulation of the polio vaccine, so I perhaps too easily took for granted the unmercenary ethic in Salk's decision not to patent the vaccine. As a result, it was quickly and cheaply mass-produced. It became available to all. I was a determined optimist: despite the terrible squander of life during the AIDS epidemic, when drug companies refused to relinquish patents in order to make palliative treatments globally affordable, I was steadfastly invested in the proposition that AIDS had taught us a lesson.

Alas, hope and reality live in different worlds. Within a year of the onset, I was asking: Why, in the face of this scourge, is there a race for patents claiming private property in vaccine development? Why is there no global sharing of research, without thought of profiting from this catastrophe? Why this setting of stakes, this competitive struggle for the property of naming and claiming? Why the planting of flags as though for colonial bragging rights? As I write this, nearly four years after the onset, I hear a news broadcast discussing the possibility that Moderna will soon raise the price of its vaccine, which will constrict its availability to poorer nations.[3]

Polio has been mostly eradicated everywhere. And the evolving potential of yet more highly effective coronavirus vaccines makes control, if not eradication, a genuine possibility. Unfortunately, widespread refusals to take vaccines at all, combined with opposition to mask wearing, have allowed new COVID variants to take hold and proliferate. The ideologically fueled rise in anti-vax sentiment has also led to a resurgence in other contagious diseases, like measles, mumps, and, yes, polio. As of January 2023, only 18 percent of U.S. adults had received a bivalent or omnivariant booster shot.[4] It does not help matters that lack of transparency and influence peddling on the part of some large profit-seeking pharmaceutical companies have eroded trust in the FDA's approval processes.[5] And so we still endure an unacceptably high rate of preventable sickness and death from COVID. What on earth has happened since the era when public-sector expertise like Jonas Salk's was trusted, respected, and revered?

As more and more of what used to be considered enmeshed social action has been restructured as personal or private decision, debates have erupted about whether shouting death threats or brandishing military-grade weapons in collective spaces is always and everywhere protected by rigidly individualized interpretations of the First Amendment. Does such behavior instead constitute an exception to free speech, like shouting fire in a crowded theater? The question of whether limits can be imposed on expressive behavior that nevertheless constrains others' freedom of political exercise by spreading fear has also been raised in the context of COVID protocols. If I am knowingly infected with COVID, choose not to wear a mask, and cough wetly on a crowded trolley—all in the name of expressing freedom of choice—is that really "nobody's business" but my own? And if a matter of public concern, are there no steps short of quarantine or imprisonment that might protect us all?

From the beginning of the pandemic until the present day, American discussions of COVID policy have been distinguished by their almost cultlike reverence for individual self-control. Strong minds would soldier through. Strong bodies would fight the enemy by denying its power or even its existence. There were undercurrents of just deserts and eugenic judgment in these discussions, as though getting sick showed a weakness of resolve: survival of the fittest became a moral proposition. These figurations were often embellished with attributes at odds with the reality of biological bodies. Imaginary incorporations drove some policies: Superman bodies, Marlboro Man bodies, steel-encased entities whose ideations were mythologized, even immortalized, as greater in importance than human epidemiological systems.

Of course, we humans are metaphor machines—to one degree or another we all believe in imaginary bodies and turn to them for strength. As a lawyer, I understand the dignity accorded to "the corpus of law." As a patriot, I respect the symbolic power of embodied national values for which soldiers in wartime would lay down their lives.

But here's what feels so unequivocally wrong: for the duration of the annus horribilis that was the year 2020, the United States was engaged in a maskless danse macabre. It was nothing less than a drawn-out, hubristic flirtation with death: a pushing of scientific limits, logical limits, ethical limits. This was neatly summarized by Texas lieutenant governor Dan Patrick: speaking of older Americans, who are statistically and immunologically more vulnerable to contracting COVID-19, he prioritized "the economy," business priorities, and "the American Dream" over the risk of dying. "There are more important things than living, and that's saving this country for my children and grandchildren."[6]

This doesn't make much sense if one believes "the country" is synonymous with "we, the people," whose lives are being sacrificed, not to an external enemy "over there," but by reason of a spreadable disease that is *in* us. The vector *is* us. This disaggregation of the country from its people and its people from a highly transmissible disease signaled an important conceptual shift in American identity. Immortalizing the economy, or perhaps capitalism, as the eternal lifeblood of our nationhood seems like a perilously fragile dream: COVID death has lowered the overall life expectancy of Americans by approximately three years, with larger drops for African Americans and Indigenous Americans. We are more than our markets. Reckless mingling in an ongoing epidemic risks much more than the economy being ruined. But if the bodies of living people are subservient or less morally important than the health of "the country" or "the economy," then perhaps the question is more about how God, country, and the economy seem to have become more embodied, more gendered, more vivacious than citizens. This reverence for "the economy" raises the question of corporate personhood.

In 1976, the Supreme Court case of *Buckley v. Valeo* held that the expenditure of money is a form of speech protected by the First Amendment.[7] The implications of that case came to an absurd and unfortunate head with the 2010 decision in *Citizens United v. Federal Elections Commission*.[8] While the *Buckley* case allows individuals unlimited spending in pursuit of political ends, *Citizens United* allows corporations that very same grace, and then some. It has created a strange sort of jurisprudence. On the one hand, corporations frequently restrict the expressions of employees or others within their purview: what they can wear, what their T-shirts can say, what political messages they can post on the walls of their offices. On the other hand, the inanimate entity of the corporation itself will now enjoy an expressive range of First Amendment benefits not limited by principles of debate or political substance, constrained only by the size of its treasury in deploying whatever technological bullhorn has the greatest chance of drowning out everyone else.

Hence, the question on many minds is why "freedom" (as in speech) has become the functional equivalent of "expenditure" (as in money); and why on earth corporations are considered "persons" to begin with.

The *Buckley* decision was controversial from the moment it was decided, for it allowed expenditures as a subcategory of the expressive power only of living individuals. A corporation, by contrast, is not only not human, it is itself property. A corporation has no natural life span, it does not vote, and many are multinational. Corporations, even nonprofits, are necessarily exclusionary, their very existence premised on bottom-line calculations, competitive power grabs, branding, prospecting for self-promotion. A corporation is legally required, by the very nature of corporate bylaws, to pursue the purpose for which it was incorporated and no other. It doesn't change its nonexistent mind or respond with compassion or feel empathy. If it does, it risks violating its internal structure, its reason for being. Thus, the "corporate citizenship" that the majority in *Citizens United* touts so blithely is a very different beast from citizenship founded on a constitution of enfranchised individuals and premised on a constituency of souls united in allegiance to an ideal of community, an egalitarianism of society, a mutual shelter of nation.

For more than a hundred years, certain inanimate entities like the corporation have been granted the status of fictive personhood for limited purposes. The concept of corporate immortality grows out of the need for a business to continue to exist despite the death of any given mortal human executive. Incorporation allows a business sufficient legal status to continue to manage assets and settle debts. When, for example, a company manufactures a defective product and sells it to you, you sue the company—not the individual officers or named employees (unless there has been some ultra vires act of extreme wrongdoing on their part, à la Richard Sackler's pushing his company's highly addictive product OxyContin, say).[9] In other words, the company is a kind of juridical stand-in for a person, with the power to sue and be sued, to make contracts, and to collect debts. This status is rooted in the efficiency interests of contract and property law, and it is extended not merely to conventional businesses, but also to such formations as municipalities, universities, law firm partnerships, etc.

All that said, it takes either the most foolish or the most cynical state of mind to conclude from this limited grant of the right to contract that therefore corporations are entitled to exactly the same panoply of civil and dignitary rights as actual, fully endowed human people (as in "We, the . . ."). The majority in *Citizens United* indulged in a skillful play of words, a suspended and suspenseful animation of humanoid endowment for corporations to express the political opinions of their principal owners by expenditure of money on behalf of political candidates. All in all, the opinion raises a big question: for whom is our Bill of Rights? Is a corporation really a "who"? Or is it a "what"? If, once upon a time, enfranchisement was calculated according to such diminishing metrics as "three-fifths of a person," doesn't this ruling confer a similar but magnifying mathematical disproportion upon the organizational prostheses we know as corporations? It is an enhancement of "person"-al power whose multiplier effect is limited only by its margin of profit.

In 1935, the great legal realist philosopher Felix Cohen wrote "Transcendental Nonsense," a wonderfully illuminating article in which he debunked (at least for that generation) the notion of corporations as literal persons.[10] Cohen challenged the reasoning of the Court of Appeals of New York in a decision about venue. The suit was brought in New York State against the Susquehanna Coal Company, a Pennsylvania corporation. In order to decide the propriety of suing in New York rather than Pennsylvania, the Court of Appeals framed the dispositive question as one of physical location: "Where is the corporation?" But as Cohen pointed out, "Nobody has ever seen a corporation. . . . What right have we to believe in corporations if we don't believe in angels? To be sure, some of us have seen corporate funds, corporate transactions, etc. (just as some of us have seen angelic deeds, angelic countenances, etc.). But this does not give us the right . . . to assume that it travels about from State to State as mortal men travel."

Cohen denounced such thinking as essentially "supernatural." He reminded jurists that a corporation does not really have a body with only one fixed "head"—that it may have a corps of employees in multiple states simultaneously:

> When the vivid fictions and metaphors of traditional jurisprudence are thought of as reasons for decisions, rather than poetical or mnemonic devices for formulating decisions reached on other grounds, then the author, as well as the reader, of the opinion or argument, is apt to forget the social forces which mold the law and the social ideals by which the law is to be judged. Thus it is that the most intelligent judges in America can deal with a concrete practical problem of procedural law and corporate responsibility without any appreciation of the economic, social, and ethical issues which it involves.[11]

In *Citizens United*, the Roberts court deployed just such a delusionary and anthropomorphizing poetical device: prosopopoeia, a figure of speech that bestows upon an abstract entity the power of speech.[12] Messieurs Snap, Crackle, and Pop, for example. The GEICO lizard. The constructive endowment that words may grant to such materially unendowed figurations is a common imaginative enterprise of the human mind. But the transference of such expressive power is always driven by, and must always be recognized as, a fiction in service to some very specific, non-imaginary end. If there is no such grounding in practical purpose, we humanize a golem. We think Mr. Clean is addressing us in real time. We hallucinate.

It helps to pay attention to and make visible the ideational bodies we have invented through such relatively common verbal gestures. In the years since the pandemic knocked us all off our feet, foggy fleets of desperate figurations have materialized as though to fill the spaces of our disorientation. Much like the Supreme Court in *Citizens United*, commentators like Dan Patrick and Glenn Beck essentially made a golem of the economy; they incorporated a mythic body to do apocalyptic battle with our fear. It's certainly understandable. COVID-19 is itself invisible, uncontrollably amorphous, so the temptation is irresistible to "see" it as an "enemy" that can be rebuffed in some material form. The yearning for control tempts us into conjuring various imaginary counterforces, benevolent specters that will stand up to the virus's murderous voraciousness.

At one point and for some, the Wall became the imagistic cure, as though steely barricades could block the dewy clouds of breath and death. Some of us prayed instead to the Winged Victory of Vaccination. Other bowed down to the Valkyries of Inherited Vitality. (In Norse mythology, Valkyrie translates as "chooser of the slain," a fierce goddess who rides bareback on her giant wolf, choosing which warriors will rise to Valhalla. The image of the Valkyrie as ruthless libertarian who grants survival to the fittest seems to have gradually displaced the generous gentility of our other civic goddesses, Blind Justice with her scales, or Lady Liberty as figured in the Statue of Liberty.)

Perhaps most powerfully of all, immunity itself has been reconfigured in some quarters as free-radical individualism—a brave and muscular man, frequently armed, with bulletproof vest and military-grade weaponry but, alas, no face mask. In 2020, Vice President Pence, impersonating this kind of warrior, faced down doctors at the Mayo Clinic, radiating strength as well as his wet breath.[13] It was, unfortunately, a colonial stance as well, whether intentional or not: if one takes a moment to acknowledge that masks are not only about protecting oneself, but also and perhaps primarily others, it ceased to look like fortitude and more like recklessness toward others.[14]

Pence later said he didn't wear masks because he wanted to look at people "in the eye."[15] Given the fact that masks don't cover the eyes, it is clear that "in the eye" meant something more than just the ocular. It referred to an aesthetic, a gaze of controlled statesmanship, to be

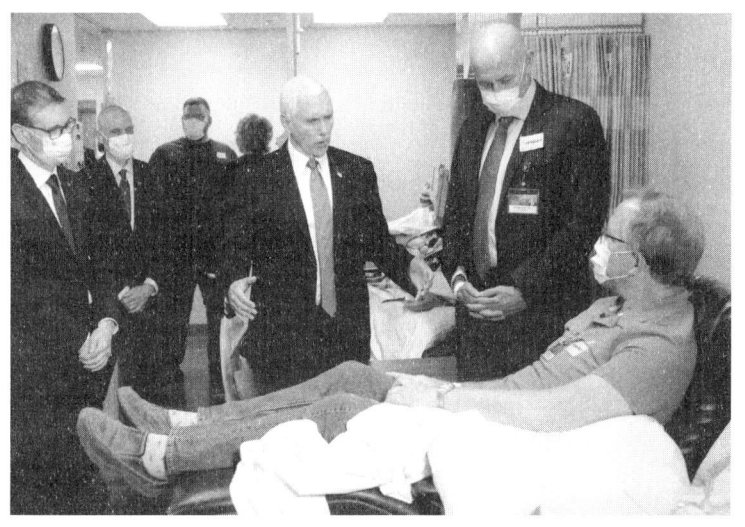

Jim Mone/AP Photo © 2020 Associated Press

read in conjunction with firmly pressed lips and a sculpturally jutting jaw, all signifying stout resolution. With a mask obstructing that profile of nose, lips, and jaw, the eyes alone become helpless, disengaged from the expressive personality of the rest of the face, so beseeching and vulnerable above the anonymity of an obliterating paper oblong. "Eye-to-eye" is a trope of masculinity, in other words, a feeling to be telegraphed, a fantasy of the strong leader who stands bare in the face of battle. Of course, it is also magical thinking, this idea of walking into the fray and dodging bullets, and emerging unscathed. It's mythmaking, a way of performing miracles. Begone coronavirus!

Perceptions of disease, deviance, and disgust have always enabled timeworn hypnotic constructions of embodied difference. When *The New Yorker* chose "The Black Plague" as a title for a really excellent piece about COVID-19 by the very insightful author Keeanga-Yahmahtta Taylor,[16] there was some pushback and rethinking of that as an unfortunate choice allowing some to think of the disease as not really affecting young white people on spring break, dancing skin to skin and partying on Florida beaches. More obviously and more powerfully, when Donald Trump (still!) speaks of "the China virus," he not only gives the disease a race and a place; true to his outsize colonial imagination, he gives it distance. It's "over there," not here, well removed from the conceptual possibility of "our" susceptibility. If "we" are afflicted, it is not just the illness that debilitates us but anger that we have been invaded by "them."

This form of displaced animus predictably provokes nativist sentiment and racial violence. There is precedent: Spikes of anti-Asian prejudice arose in the wake of outbreaks of smallpox in San Francisco's Chinatown in the 1800s; they culminated in the Chinese Exclusion Act of 1882.[17] Anti-Semitic nativism targeted Jews after bouts of typhus in 1892.[18] Mary Mallon, or "Typhoid Mary," was an asymptomatic carrier of typhoid fever; her arrest in 1907 on public health charges galvanized much anti-Irish sentiment in New York City, figuring them as immigrants importing unsanitary and slovenly habits.[19] When the AIDS epidemic first started spreading in the 1980s, some people told themselves it was a disease conveniently localized to the bodies of "gay men." And when Zika virus was carried from equatorial regions by mosquitoes riding the waves of climate change, New York City health officials sprayed insecticide by zip code (focusing on East Flatbush, Bedford-Stuyvesant, Crown Heights, and Brownsville in Brooklyn, and on the neighborhood once known as Spanish Harlem in upper Manhattan) as though those pesky identity-politicking mosquitoes could simply be redlined.[20]

Instead of coming together around our shared vulnerability, time and again we have created a set of scapegoats to stand in for a pathogen, divisive demons that direct our fears of inherent virulence, murderous voraciousness, and parasitism. Asians. "Aliens." People who wear masks. People who don't wear masks. Peaceful demonstrators transformed into the face of "corona violence." It is not by accident that former president Trump's 2020 campaign ads targeted "white suburban housewives"; the ads neatly sutured race, riot, and disease as a way to channel the existential fear to which we are all so vulnerable right now: if you can keep "them" out of your neighborhood, everything is going to be all right.

Collectively, we Americans seem not now inclined to believe in the entanglements of a common fate. The very notion of public health has been undermined by ingrained brands of individualism so radical that even contagious disease is officially regulated by the vocabulary of "choice," "freedom," and "personal responsibility." Many of us live in bubbles of belief that conceptual walls will protect us from things that are not easily walled: guns will bring peace; housing discrimination will bring bliss to soccer moms; segregated schools will serve up stable geniuses; and owning an island in the Florida Keys will seal us off from child molesters, mafia dons, and domestic abuse.

These comforting bromides set us up for naive beliefs that disease invariably marks bodies in visible ways.

"Surely we'll be able to see it coming."

"You're fine if you don't have a fever."

"You can't spread it if you're not coughing."

"You won't give it to anyone if you're asymptomatic."

Well before this pandemic, we were blinded by the walls of our privatized bunkers, yet the sense of entitlement that supposes disaster will strike "over there" but "not in my backyard" pretty much guarantees an amplification of misdirected resources and relative disparities from which everyone will suffer eventually.

One of the most difficult challenges in a time of moral panic is undoing such a profound confusion of terms. To understand the true dimension of that problem, it helps to look at the document that most succinctly captures the thinking behind federal COVID policy as pursued during most of the year 2020: the Great Barrington Declaration.[21] Although it was not officially published until October of that year, it summarized the thinking of the Trump administration's most hyper-libertarian advisors, including Dr. Scott Atlas, and then secretary of Health and Human Services Alex Azar. The authors, a loose collective of epidemiologists and doctors, were proponents of a strategy they called Focused Protection. They asserted that "current lockdown policies" were causing "irreparable damage, with the underprivileged disproportionately harmed." It is worth noticing that in this version of reality, the more active agent of such harm is not the actual virus, but "lockdown." The expressed goal of the authors was "reaching herd immunity" by opening up everything—*everything*, period—and soldiering through. According to them, literally encouraging community spread would supposedly "allow those who are at minimal risk of death to live their lives normally to build up immunity to the virus through natural infection, while better protecting those who are at highest risk." Sunetra Gupta, one of the three principal authors, told *The Daily Telegraph*: "We're saying, let's just do this for the three months it takes for the pathogen to sweep through the population."[22] And Martin Kulldorff, another principal author, told Canada's *National Post* what he envisioned: "Anybody above 60, whether teacher or bus driver or janitor I think should not be working—if those in their 60s can't work from home they should be able to take a sabbatical (supported by Social Security) for three, four, or whatever months it takes before there is immunity in the community that will protect everybody."[23]

Innumerable ethical questions are raised by such a proposition, not least its unproved assumption that the human population was anywhere near the happy status of "building up" immunity. The rise and proliferation of new, more transmissible variants seems not to have been given a thought; and the enduring disabilities inflicted by long COVID were seriously underestimated. Then too, there was the thoughtlessly impractical description of what "better protection" for those at higher risk would look like: "Nursing home staff should use staff with acquired immunity"—as though there's a workforce of the certifiably immune just waiting to be hired.

Even though vaccines have proved very effective, their slow, chaotic rollout at the start created distrust, and policymakers under the sway of the Declaration were committed to the assumption that "acquired immunity" would be a cheaper option than actual preparation for mass production and distribution of vaccines, to say nothing of sufficient personal protective equipment (PPE). The declaration also asserted that "Retired people living at home should have groceries and other essentials delivered to their home. When possible, they should meet family members outside rather than inside"[24]—as though there's a world in which "retired" people come neatly segregated in separate homes, apart from non-retired family. Even the use of the term "retired" as a cipher for age seemed to focus on those no longer contributing to the economy; it skirted around the degree to which many people over the age of sixty-five have to keep working because Social Security does not cover the costs of living, even before the pandemic became a factor.

One of the most appalling aspects of the declaration was its substitution of the term "herd immunity" for the "community spread" it was actually proposing. Herd immunity more accurately refers to a contagion against which there has been made available widespread programs of vaccination—typically vaccination rates of between 60 and 80 percent of a population.[25] That in turn depends upon the existence of a scientifically efficacious vaccine that ensures immunity for a stable and significant period of time. In contrast, the term "community spread" captures the promiscuous, relentless virality of infectious disease.[26] We may have herd immunity (or "herd mentality," as Trump misstated it),[27] and we certainly have spread. But we have nothing close to immunity.

Moreover, it is far from clear whether infection guarantees immunity, or for how long. As has been obvious from endless spikes among partying college students and professional athletes, the young and the buff are more susceptible than the Great Barrington Declaration allows, and even if they seem to represent a lesser proportion of immediate fatalities, they may suffer disproportionately from long-term cardiopulmonary syndromes and disabling vascular disorders.[28] Most perniciously, the Great Barrington Declaration ignores altogether the reality that COVID-19 may be spread by those with no outward or visible symptoms. Its authors make no mention of the need for widespread, repeated, reliable testing of the asymptomatic.

By these confusingly compressed definitions, "herd immunity" would require that 60 to 80 percent of a given population not only have been "exposed," but have recovered sufficiently to have developed antibodies—around 200 million Americans. (As of March 2021, there had been about 30 million American cases since the onset in March of 2020, or less than 10 percent of the U.S. population.) Only at those levels would unvaccinated vulnerable people have a hope of being protected. Again, the Great Barrington Declaration did not propose that herd immunity happen through vaccination. Its suggestion that those levels be acquired "naturally" refers to those left standing after untold greater calamity: first, those for whom exposure does not result in death; second, those who sufficiently recover to have developed enduring antibodies; and third, those not left with long-term or permanent disability. To get to that point without a vaccine means tolerating many more deaths—not to mention violently destabilizing rates of grave and protracted illness. As intentional policy, this ends up not looking like "survival," even of the fittest; it looks like an intentionally induced avalanche of slaughter.

Moreover, the propagation of such deadly confusion was assisted by deeply contested hierarchies of legitimacy and a jabbering bewilderment of competing sources, all laying claim to "truth." Although the Great Barrington Declaration claimed to be endorsed by tens of thousands of medical professionals, the vetting of signatories lacked rigor (hence, endorsements from such eminent authorities as "Dr. Johnny Bananas" and "Dr. Person Fakename").[29] In short, it is a crowdsourced ideological tract sponsored by the American Institute of Economic Research, a libertarian umbrella group located in Great Barrington, Massachusetts, which adheres to Austrian School economic notions of methodological individualism. Major donors include Charles Koch and the Bradley J. Madden Foundation, which has worked to evade and erode the FDA's regulatory mechanisms and processes designed to ensure health and safety protections in the approval of new drugs and vaccines.

The institute's other sponsored tracts include titles like "Brazilians Should Keep Slashing Their Rainforest." Consider a post on the institute's website written by one of its research fellows, John Tamny (also editor of RealClearMarkets.com), "Imagine If the Virus Had Never Been Detected." He asserted that:

> The coronavirus is a rich man's virus. . . . People live longer today, and they do because major healthcare advances born of wealth creation made living longer possible. We wouldn't have noticed this virus 100 years ago. We weren't rich enough. . . . What is most lethal to older people isn't much noticed by those who aren't old. A rapidly spreading virus was seemingly not much of a factor until politicians needlessly made it one. . . . The virus didn't suddenly start spreading in March of 2020 just because politicians decided it had. The likelier beginning is 2019. Early 2020 too. Life was pretty normal as a virus made its way around the world then. Politicians made it abnormal. Let's never forget the sickening carnage they can create when they find reasons to "do something."[30]

Let me underscore that this post was dated *February 4, 2021*, during a a week in which there were 21,000 COVID deaths in the United States alone.[31] Worldwide, 2021 was the deadliest year of the pandemic, with COVID rising to the leading cause of death in most countries, accountable for at least 3.9 million deaths worldwide.[32]

Unsurprisingly, the glib, laissez-faire recommendations of the Great Barrington Declaration were opposed by an overwhelming consensus of public health experts, including the NIH, the CDC, the World Health Organization, the Mayo Clinic, and Johns Hopkins Medical School, as well as globally regarded scientists, including Drs. Anthony Fauci and Francis Collins.

All that said, the Great Barrington Declaration became dark reality because its free-market strategies have been embraced at the highest levels of American governance and businesses, mirroring what has happened in the past with other powerful lobbying interests, such as the tobacco and lead paint industries. This stance was aligned not only with Ayn Randian ultra-libertarianism, but also became entangled with the sovereign-citizen movement—militant anti-mask, anti-vaxxers willing to take up arms to resist stay-at-home guidelines; belligerent anti-government souls whose extremism inspires them to descend upon legislatures in bids to ensure we may all live to die for a free-market economy.

This convergence of anti-regulatory sentiments meant not only that the pandemic continued to rip through certain vulnerable populations, but also that the tragedy of such massive loss will imprint itself upon us as enduring collective trauma. And at a moment when fact sometimes seems to have been locked behind an inscrutable cosmic paywall, the bipartisan angst emerging from a national sense of siege should not be underestimated as its own governing force. This is an altogether dreadful moment. And dread eludes logic or law or rational discourse; it is powerfully destabilizing as well as powerfully directive.

Yet the Great Barrington Declaration promised: "A comprehensive and detailed list of measures, including approaches to multigenerational households, can be implemented, and is well within the scope and capability of public health professionals." But to a hungrily contagious virus, any in-person mingling—school, bar, gym, office—is the absolute equivalent of a "multigenerational household." This reality of unbounded human sociality is, of course, the crux of the problem, and precisely what's missing from the declaration's analysis—as well as from both the Trump and Biden administrations' responses: If there is such a "list of measures," we should have had it posted on every public billboard long ago. Instead, tracking the real incidence of COVID has become nearly impossible, because public testing sites have been dismantled and collection of data has been individualized via a casual opt-in deployment of "self-testing" kits. With undercounting thus almost guaranteed, we nevertheless know for certain that as of early 2023, more than a million Americans have died from COVID. And although we have reached the declaration's "herd immunity" goal of having about 200 million people infected, as of mid-2023 there are still at least a hundred thousand new cases a week, and deaths average around two thousand a week.[33]

Despite all this, in September 2022, President Biden, in an interview on *60 Minutes*, confidently declared that "the pandemic is over."[34] I was startled by the substantive thinness of the claim, but to my ear it also sounded like an expedient overstatement common in the determined optimism of political speech. It made me think of George W. Bush standing in front of that banner MISSION ACCOMPLISHED— when the woe in Iraq had barely begun. It made me think of pundits who described Barack Obama's election as proof that "We are post-racial!" It's a peculiarly American habit of diction, to turn the subjunctive mood into the present tense, imbuing it with truth. I think of it as the Wishful Immediate. Not quite a lie, it nonetheless turns a hypothetical into ontological existence. It takes the "might" of a future possibility, strips away the contingencies, and serves it up as an irrefutably present thing.

The diction of the American Dream—*You can be anything you put your mind to*—is also the diction of contract law: it takes expectation interests and turns them into prospects that can be treated as present phenomena. *I don't need masks or vaccines because I am right-thinking. Think rightly for yourself and you won't be vulnerable either!* It's the legal fiction that allows us to have credit and futures markets. It works well as a prompt for transactors to throw themselves into a future moment as though it were the present, to bring a wish, a desired outcome, into fruition. It's why we call it the expectation theory of contract, or "will" theory. Desires are honored as palpable and worthy in the present tense. All things are possible, all probabilities are present, all fantasies made real. You didn't just wish it were so, it *was*. The present imaginary rewrites the past.

In the context of a public health emergency like COVID, however, this optimistic presentism sometimes invites us to confuse the American dream of a cornucopic national body with individual states of health. To acknowledge one's mortal vulnerability is to betray the nation. This is perhaps symptomatic of a national mood that routinely considers itself only a purchase away from perfection. The American work ethic that for so long promised "anything" as possible has morphed into a wish ethic that tolerates no earthly limit. It is a greedy state of mind, and I worry that it almost structures us to allow dissembling as a kind of blind ambition. We need some consciousness about what we are doing when we confuse what we want with what is. Otherwise, this conceptual conflation divides us from history, from facts, from sinkholes in the road of life, and floats us gently into Wonderland.

5
Utopia

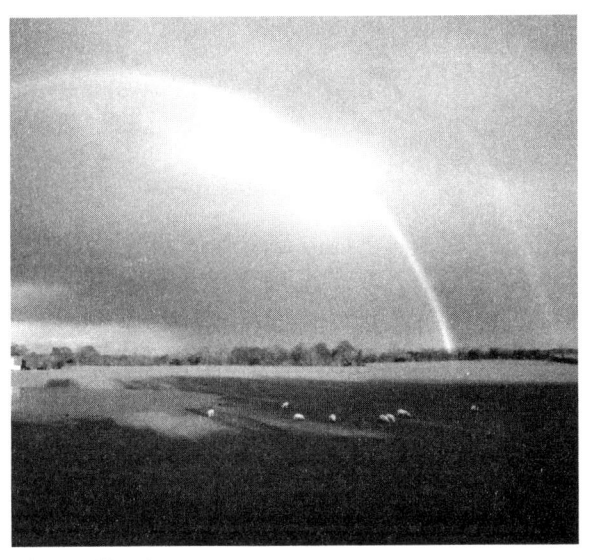

mikeroman6/Getty Images

A few years ago, I drove through Goodyear, Arizona, a town founded in 1917 by the Goodyear rubber company as a location to grow cotton for use in the webbing with which early tires were cohered.[1] The cotton fields are still there, an odd sight in the middle of the Sonoran Desert. My journey through Goodyear coincided with a rainstorm. As the clouds cleared, a glorious double rainbow arced in a complete semicircle from one side of the horizon to the other.

Awed, I pulled to the side of the road to look. Just then, a Goodyear blimp floated by on a trajectory as though to sail beneath the rainbow in supreme aeronautical triumphalism. Note, too, that the end of the rainbow has landed its lucky pot o' gold smack-dab upon a brand-new Amazon Distribution Center being built in the middle of this beautiful chaparral, until recently a spot apparently known to locals as "the middle of nowhere." Despite its odd mash-up of nature and industry, the panorama was beautiful—utopic even. Still, I was left wondering: Does working in "the middle of "nowhere" mark a worker as "nobody"?

This took place in 2019, just before COVID-19 made economic crisis the lens through which all labor would be interrogated for its value to the national economy. Physical, on-site employment of all sorts—package handling, food processing, delivery services, mechanical engineering, nursing, etc.—was scrutinized to determine which work should be considered "necessary," and which workers deemed "essential."[2]

It's worth underscoring the distinction between *necessary work* and *essential workers* in sorting out moral agency and legal obligations. Historically, the category of essential worker emphasizes what is essential for protecting national security infrastructure. In executive orders issued by presidents Trump and Biden, essential workers are defined in relation to Homeland Security: workers in the fields of medicine, health care, policing, transportation, agriculture and food supply chains, water, communications, energy supply, and finance systems.[3] So demarcated, essential workers are those whose autonomy is then constrained by duty and obligation to a higher calling, to wit, protection of collective interest in the integrity of the national security infrastructure. These essential laborers are required to respond, somewhat like the draft, to a public calling that may require laying down one's own life for a collective cause, the life of the nation—which, like the flag, is conceptualized as a living thing. (Little as it's known, the United States Flag Code says "The flag represents a living country and is itself considered a living thing."[4] It's why flag pins are worn over the heart, or on the left side of the body.) There's something heroic, even religious when work is framed as that sort of sacrifice.

However, there are affective differences intuitively envisioned with those categories. We all share images of the heroic doctors, nurses, police officers, truckers, bankers, and communications experts who labor to keep us together in ways we applaud and thank. In contrast, we have shown very little recognition of meatpackers, janitors, sewage workers, and gravediggers—jobs that, in normal times, many deem "peripheral." Peripheral realms of labor tend not to summon images of sacrifice. And even though farmworkers and meatpackers are grouped with bankers and doctors as "essential workers," those industries exist in different referential universes. Hence, discussions of peripheral labor tend to shift in focus away from essential *workers* to necessary *work*. The discourse shifts from a constitutionally relational holiness of "we who serve," to a narrower focus on work to be done. The work becomes a thing. Manufacture and production thus become abstracted and disembodied from the persons who render the thing.

In other words, as we shift our reference from essential workers to necessary work, we shift from people to production. We shift from a basic aim of reducing suffering and death to a different aim, one of supply, with emphasis on the products that allow a certain standard of living to purchasers, consumers. We want enough beef and toilet paper as drivers of the economy. We want the work as product, without any particular focus on the labor of work*ers*.

Consider Upton Sinclair's great American novel *The Jungle*, written in 1906, about the deplorable practices of the meatpacking industry in Chicago, which Jack London labeled the "*Uncle Tom's Cabin* of wage slavery."[5] Sinclair was a socialist, and he wrote the book to decry the dismally corrupt and exploitative working conditions in the stockyards, and the dire treatment of immigrant workers, largely from Ireland and Eastern Europe. There's a passage in the book that became a flashpoint for the reading public: workers fall into the rendering vats and are ground up and processed along with animal parts, only to be packaged and sold as "Durham's Pure Leaf Lard." That scene became the emotional hook for the book's success and shifted public outcry from labor conditions of immigrant workers to product safety for the consuming public. As Sinclair himself acknowledged, the book succeeded "not because the public cared anything about the workers, but simply because the public did not want to eat tubercular beef." That outcry led to the official start of the regulatory state in America, when the administration of Theodore Roosevelt passed the Meat Inspection Act, The Pure Food and Drug Act, and the Bureau of Chemistry, later renamed the Food and Drug Administration.[6]

I mention all this as antecedent to our current condition, where one of the industries in which there's been the greatest neglect and controversy about wretched pandemic working conditions is—yes, the meatpacking industry. The workforce consists primarily of recent migrants from south of the border, large numbers of whom are undocumented and unable to complain. Working conditions in meatpacking have always been dreadful, but they were made worse during the pandemic by lack of personal protective equipment, the lack of sick leave, and assembly lines that pack people together with no distancing. COVID death rates in these jobs—largely among people of color and women—are huge. Indeed, Blacks and Latinos, disproportionately employed as low-level peripheral laborers have constituted as much as 43 percent of all deaths from COVID-19, although together they represent under 30 percent of the U.S. population.[7] In effect, the employment and living conditions of people of color are as important mortality risks as age. Dr. Uché Blackstock, CEO of Advancing Health Equity, observes: "It's almost as if living in a country with racism ages people . . . to the point where even people who are not elderly . . . are still susceptible to dying from this virus in a way that's very similar to people who are elderly."[8]

These long-standing health care disparities afflicting racial minorities have been incalculably exacerbated by policies of neglect. Nor is this catastrophe merely one of unequal health outcomes: the fallout includes disproportionate debt, job loss, homelessness, educational deficits, child welfare fiascoes, trauma, and grief. The cascading consequences of such social disruption have been one of the greatest legacies of the pandemic.

I used to teach a course on agricultural laws governing the treatment of animals—the handling of meat products, the poultry laws, the ovine and porcine caging requirements, regulations dictating the conditions of benevolent slaughter. In the wake of COVID, those laws sometimes seem to provide more protection than do OSHA protections for workers in the abattoirs. Our system of Occupational Safety and Health puts workers in an untenable bargaining position when they seek labor reform or claim recompense for illness caused by working conditions.[9] First, OSHA requires that sickness must take place "on the job"— virtually impossible to prove in a pandemic. It casts workers as discrete agents, as atomized units, and it treats the workplace as nonporous when it comes to contagious disease. Under Worker's Compensation laws, too, workers have to prove they've been infected on the job. It is not a construct that deals with the reality of epidemic or contagion. Even the Emergency Paid Sick Leave Act doesn't apply to operations with more than five hundred or fewer than fifty employees.[10]

This construct of a purely private worksite sealed off from public governance or interest flows from the contractarian logic whereby factory interiors are governed by broad notions of "at will" employment: *Leave if you don't like it.* Community and its contagions exist beyond those walls of "personal preference." To make matters worse, OSHA was already the most underfunded it had ever been before the pandemic began; President Trump slashed the number of inspectors by another 8 percent the moment he took office.[11] Furthermore, it's been up to states how to make OSHA's advice and guidance mandatory; unsurprisingly, states have produced a vast checkerboard of requirements and a vast inconsistency of political nattering.

If public health is seen through the metrics of the factory interior, where everything operates according to laissez-faire notions, it can be seen as threatening to manufacturing interests. From this perspective, the assertion of public health is often cast as a response that not only federalizes but "nationalizes" worker health and safety. (Private industries often hurl accusations of "socialism" at this point in labor discussions.) Indeed, even as numbers of COVID deaths mounted, industries of all sorts—from meatpackers to airlines—marshaled well-funded attacks upon regulatory requirements regarding workplace safety, vaccines, masks, and other protective gear. The most effective of these attacks have manipulated discourse as well: to wit, supplanting constitutional language of common good with the language of hyper-libertarianism and sovereign identitarianism. For example, anti-masking could be expressed as an industrialist's dream: businesses "don't have to" provide masks or other protection because it's the workers who don't want to be told what to do. It's their choice!

Moreover, this way of thinking becomes internalized even by those for whom it is against some degree of self-interest. If I were suffering from a virulently contagious pathogen, one way of discussing my status could certainly be that such affliction is "all about me." If I adhere to a rigid measure of individual contract and freedom of choice, I could also decide that my condition is "nobody's business but my own," and that the rest of the world should just let me be. It becomes hard to think beyond such binarism, to hold two ideas in one's head at the same time, to recognize the complexity that contagious illness is a communal affliction as much as an individual one. If I decide to go to my job as a cook in a restaurant or to take a crowded bus to visit my aunt in a nursing home, the morality of my action becomes more vexed as a matter of social, public, and constitutional interest. Similarly, if the medication used to treat my disease is developed, owned, patented, or licensed by a single company, it will be worrying if the company treats me as just another contractor in a perfectly free market rather than as a patient whose life is in their hands. It will be worrying if it charges me a sky-high price governed by no limit other than the highest bidder and the profit interest of its shareholders. For these reasons, it makes a big difference if the medication is developed or governed by a nonprofit public health infrastructure whose ethical interest is in distributing the greatest good for the greatest number, thereby constraining the epidemiology of harm that implicates the fate of me as well as multitudes.

Nor is it just business profit underwriting the extreme libertarianism of this time. There's also that seductive myth of volitionally assumed suicidality that *chooses* death—not on behalf of our common identity as citizens or our common humanity, but as part of a survival-of-the-fittest narrative. Survival of the fittest is, in turn, entangled with all sorts of other myths about labor, the rational economic actor, model minorities, and immigrants who don't complain because they *want* to work hard, harder, hardest. Myths about immigrants who *want* to do the work that real Americans won't do. Myths about dark people and immigrants being inherently physically stronger because of supposed biological endowment. Myths about backbreaking work and lousy conditions being good for moral fiber. Myths about hard work making aliens less alien and possibly more white. Myths teaching that no matter how dangerous or unfair the working conditions here, it's better than the "shithole" countries from whence they emanated. *They're lucky to be here.*

As in Sinclair's observations about conditions in 1906, sick and mistreated employees are treated as cogs in a machine. Now, as then, there are two problems: first, the human labor problem, and second, the meatpacking industry's lack of fiduciary relationship to the public's interest in the fair trade of safe goods. But one becomes conflated with the other in terms of regulatory priority. And to this day, we see a much too comfortable shift in our priorities away from the health, safety, and welfare of people imprisoned by the near-impossible working conditions imposed by catastrophic global crises. Instead, we take comfort in the contract justifications of "choosing" one's own lot in life—of literally putting one's body on the line—cast as a volitional choice. As in 1906, we turn away from the basic health of *workers* to attend to the need for contract fulfillment of desired *production* goals: gas prices, eggs, the availability of computer chips, and whether there will be another Super Bowl run on chicken wings, avocados, and toilet paper.

6
Making Nice

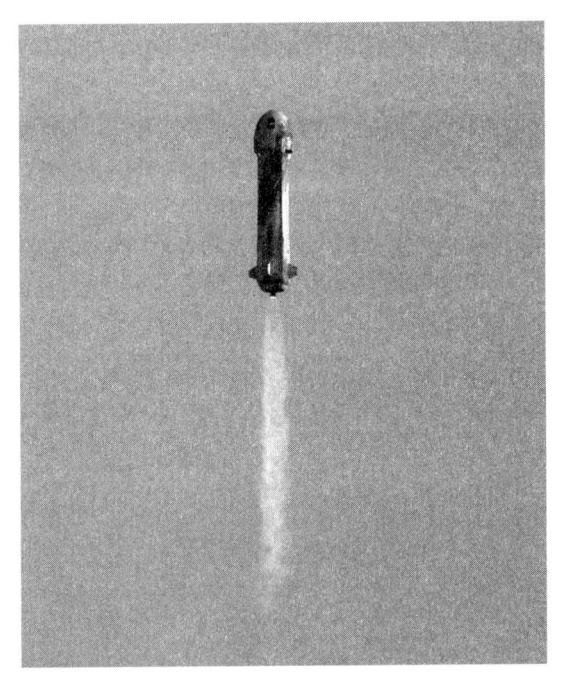

Joe Raedle/Getty Images

One very conspicuous difference between the framework of the Great Barrington Declaration about COVID herd immunity, and Jonas Salk's life-affirming generosity in not patenting the polio vaccine is the underlying story we tell ourselves about the efficacy of res publicae and a shared commons. It is not just that public-sector budgets in America have been progressively and intentionally starved at every level. There has also been a massive discursive shift away from the language of public enterprise and toward the enunciations of private entrepreneurialism. Just compare the (perhaps apocryphal) words Neil Armstrong uttered at the first moon landing in 1969: "That's one small step for man, one giant leap for mankind."[1] It was memorable for its generosity of referential regard—it was a celebration of planetary relation. Contrast that to the words uttered in 2021 by actor William Shatner to billionaire Jeff Bezos after privately purchasing a ten-minute ride in Bezos's dildo-shaped spaceship: "What you've given me is the most profound experience I can imagine."[2]

Shatner also said, "This is now the commercial: it would be so important for everyone to have that experience through one means or anything—maybe you put it on 3D and wear goggles to have that experience." Like Shannon Whisnant, who bought John Woods's leg, Shatner boiled things down to a "you-me" exchange, a "commercial" opportunity, and a fungible "experience" to boot. This was the language of a private individual speaking to his lord benefactor monopoly techno-king. Captain Kirk had gone to "like-Disneyland."

The transformation from a global world of "we" to the privacy of Shatner and Bezos's individualized exchange depends on particular ideological constructions of the body. I am my own person when expressing an odd preference for what I wish to eat for dinner. I am less "my own" and more of a social actor if I "choose" to throw dead dogs into the community well. And even the staunchest individualists become fluid in their identity when someone runs through a mall shooting people. In such moments of desperate alarm, our vulnerability equalizes us, if only somewhat. This latter underscores the fluidity by which we can be singular for some purposes but simultaneously entangled as members of a social body whose health we protect by collective preparedness (beforehand) and imposition of criminal law (after the fact).

Different bodies of law frame liability around each of these constructions: for example, in contract laws, an atomized *Homo economicus* of a body is imagined as accountable to no one but those with whom he has *voluntarily agreed* to contract. In constitutional law, a citizen body is imagined to be porously interconnected with multiple systems of policy, sustenance, and obligation (whether imposed or voluntarily undertaken). Ideally, we temper our law and its varied imaginaries according to circumstance and norms of harmony—like a slide trombone seeking the perfect note. The law grants great autonomy to the woman who loves burnt toast and fish eyes for dinner; we, society, back off because dinner is appropriately deemed a private realm, her very own Principality of Hutt. But the law considers the same woman a piece and a part of a larger social body when she enters a synagogue and spews anti-Semitic epithets. At least that's conceptually how the law has been understood until rather recently. Recently that zone of contract choice, privacy, and individual right has been increasingly transformed into more and more of an impermeably walled geography of antisociality—ultra-libertarianism, stuck on one rigidly defined note, with no sliding scale of relational harmony or constitutive community.

For one example of this discursive shift, the First Amendment's protection of free speech has been increasingly fused with the Second Amendment's right to bear arms. In the 2008 case of *District of Columbia v. Heller*,[3] the Supreme Court de-linked the Second Amendment's right to bear arms from the maintenance of a well-regulated militia; with that decision, assembling an armamentarium of military-grade weaponry became a personal expressive right. The crisis that such an expansive ruling has engendered for both "individual freedom" and "personal expression" is perfectly captured by an increasing number of incidents that test the limits of law itself: In Missouri, a man carrying a loaded AR-style rifle, a handgun, and a hundred rounds of ammunition walked into a Walmart grocery store, while recording himself with a camera. Panic ensued, and he was held by an off-duty fireman who was carrying a gun of his own. "I wanted to see if that Walmart honored the Second Amendment," the culprit told police after he was arrested on second-degree terrorism charges. The prosecutor couldn't charge him for any gun-related violation, so he relied on a law making it illegal to "knowingly communicate an implied threat to cause an incident or condition involving danger to life or cause fear that a condition existed involving danger to life."[4] After all, forty-seven out of fifty states allow for open carry of handguns or long arms or both. In Texas a man was arrested as he approached a dance hall wearing a spiked leather face mask while carrying an AR-15 and a Bible. Under Texas's lenient gun laws, all he could be charged with was the misdemeanor of disorderly conduct, which includes displaying a firearm "in a manner calculated to alarm." Recently, a man was arrested after going into a Publix grocery store in Atlanta, Georgia, wearing antiballistic armor and carrying four handguns, a semiautomatic rifle, and a 12-gauge shotgun. Here is a photo of the guns the man carried into that supermarket:

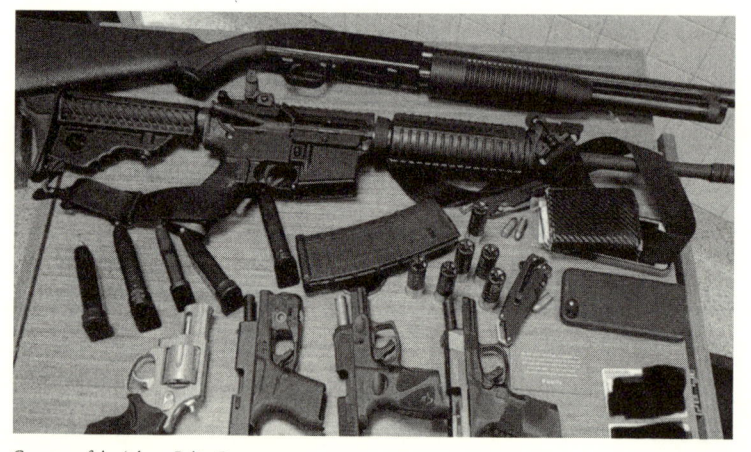

Courtesy of the Atlanta Police Department

The man's defense lawyer challenged his arrest, asking: "What is the definition of reckless conduct? Carrying weapons? In a state that requires no permit? And no license? I mean, help me understand, what's the reckless conduct?"[5]

Indeed, it's hard to distinguish what a sane resolution to this might be when lawmakers themselves model aggressively bellicose forms of public encounter. This is Kentucky Congressman Thomas Massie's Christmas card from 2021:[6]

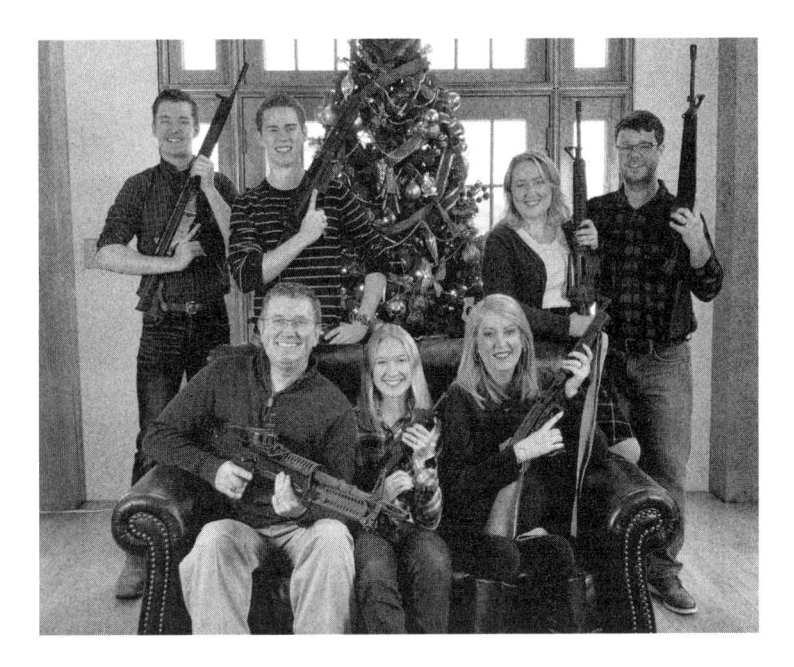

Similarly, Congresswoman Lauren Boebert's 2021 holiday card featured her four young sons, ranging in age from about 8 to 15, each happily bearing his own enormous assault rifle.

Until recently, extrajudicial killing was presumptively the realm of criminality. But of late, the notion that one's own family can legitimately act as a private army has underwritten the proliferation of ever more expansive notions of "self-defense" and access to weaponry. It is surely a vexed time, weighted with foreboding, anxiety, and grief. We are all afraid of something: terrorism, random outlaws with PTSD, ominous political forces. As a result, gun sales have soared. Paradoxically, rising gun sales mean that police become edgier, more afraid, and more likely to literally "jump the gun" in a climate where anyone and everyone may be armed. Nevertheless, warns Ted Shaw, director of the Center for Civil Rights at the University of North Carolina and former director of the NAACP Legal Defense Fund, referring to cases like Philando Castile's, "in a society that worships gun culture and advocates the right to carry weapons, it cannot be that the fact that an individual has a gun automatically justifies shooting him."

On the other hand, the history of the right to bear arms has been shaped by exclusionary privilege based on race and gender. It is almost exclusively white men who may "reasonably" carry firearms to protests outside supermarkets or polling places or political conventions. It is almost exclusively white men who do not need to retreat from domestic disputes while on ground deemed "theirs." Nonwhites and women, however, are much less likely to be able to walk through the world with assault rifles (or toy guns, or the shadow of anything that might resemble a gun) and not be mowed down for that reason alone—either by police or the idealized citizen-savior.

In her book *Stand Your Ground: A History of America's Love Affair with Lethal Self-Defense*, Harvard professor Caroline Light traces the history of our romance with legalized vigilantism. She dates it to the Reconstruction era, "when post-war political and economic turmoil and the enfranchisement of African-American men fed late-19th-century gender panic, and the legal terrain shifted to characterize a man's 'castle' and the dependents residing therein as an extension of the white masculine self." Light asserts that current policies, including defunding basic public services, have led to a situation in which "the state's retreat from the protection of its citizens creates a perceived need for (do-it-your) self-defense." The supposedly race-neutral idea of "reasonable threat" actually encourages a "lethal response to Black intrusions into spaces considered white."[7]

Recently, an officer from the North Miami Police Department shot and wounded Charles Kinsey, a Black therapist trying to help a severely autistic patient who had wandered away from a mental-health

Making Nice 77

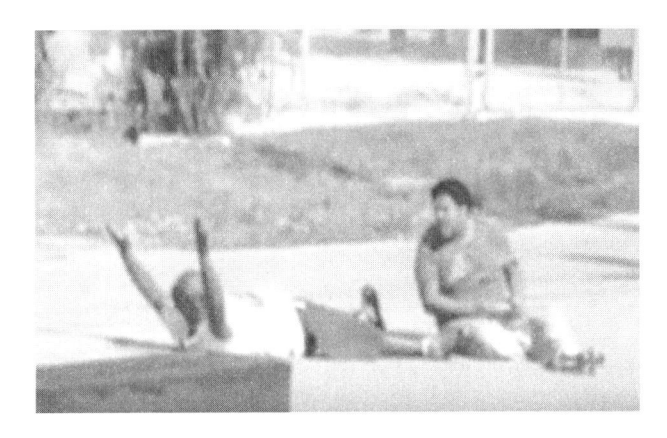

center and into traffic. Pictures taken by passersby showed that neither the patient nor Kinsey was armed. Indeed, Kinsey had identified himself, explained the situation, and was lying on the ground with his hands in the air when the police shot him.

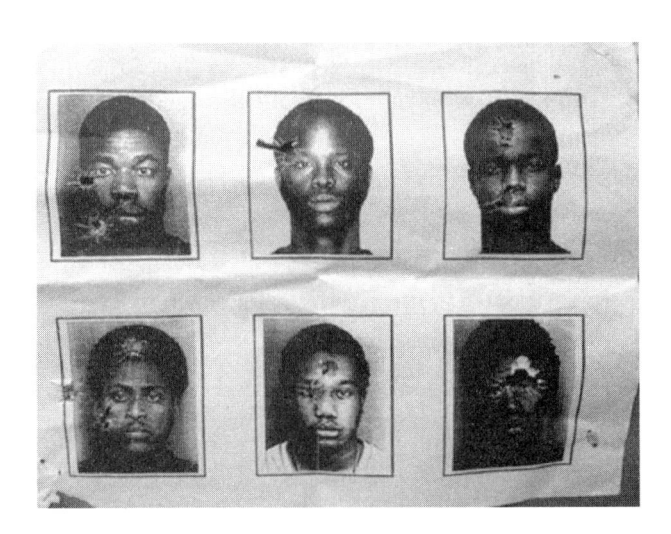

When asked later why he had shot Kinsey, the officer who pulled the trigger replied, "I don't know." Such a twitchy hair-trigger response reminded me that the North Miami Police Department had been chastised just the year before for using mug shots of African American arrestees for target practice.[8] It is hard to discount the possibility that such "practice" might successfully train the eye toward what to fear and whom to kill.

Against this already charged backdrop, a circuit judge in Broward County, Florida, recently extended Florida's "stand your ground" law to protect police officers.[9] The case at issue involved the 2013 death of Jermaine McBean, a thirty-three-year-old Black man who was shot three times after being spotted walking on a busy street carrying what turned out to be an unloaded Airsoft rifle. The judge dismissed all criminal charges against Broward County Sheriff's Deputy Peter Peraza, based on his assertion that he had no duty to retreat because he believed that McBean was trying to kill or seriously harm him.[10]

Stand-your-ground laws are a subspecies of self-defense. The idea is that "ground" is jurisprudentially defined as a space from which one has the reasonable expectation of excluding others—i.e., one's property. What makes the idea of standing one's ground so troubling is precisely the question of whose ground it is anyway—yours or mine? What, indeed, of "our" ground? Law enforcement officers, after all, are charged with a duty to serve and protect public, collective geographies, not just "their" ground.

Stand-your-ground laws have extended the older defense of one's "castle" beyond the walls of one's home to one's individual and subjectively determined comfort zone. This, in effect, allows a public street to be turned into conceptually private space. However problematic this may be in citizen encounters, judging police by this measure represents a seismic shift in accountability. It is a cornerstone of our legal system—and of international law—that police, as state actors, respond to objective standards, not subjective emotions. Our expectation is that they will be well-trained in techniques of defusing confrontation, and that they will deploy force only as a last resort. If, instead, the mere experience of fear justifies violence anyplace, anytime, we have set a dangerous precedent regardless of race, gender, or occupation—

but especially in the case of police. There is a tension between the call of duty—which is one of public service, even self-sacrifice—and the unmoored fears harbored by those who don't know anyone in the neighborhoods they're assigned to patrol. There are at least some who, in the absence of training, experience, self-restraint, and proper support, may fill that void with assumptions and panic—who would place self-protection so far ahead of the duty to protect the community that they succumb much too easily to an ethic of "Shoot first, ask questions later."

Unfortunately, in lieu of any serious political discussion about gun control, there has been instead a proliferation of laws and bills that would further privatize public safety, by arming schoolteachers and training them to kill.[11] Observes Adam Skaggs, of the Giffords Law Center to Prevent Gun Violence, "It's the idea that people need guns everywhere—city streets, public parks, even government buildings."[12] It's also the response of a nation at war with itself. One example of the trend is the Buckeye Firearms Foundation's funding of so-called Faster programs, three-day gun training sessions for teachers from around the country.[13] In addition to target practice, one day of the training is devoted to "mindset development," or bolstering teachers' preparedness to shoot after split-second assessments. Trainees are asked "to close their eyes and imagine the student entering the classroom with a gun" and then are taught how to command the grit necessary to kill that student. One teacher from Colorado told the BBC that "she decided to picture her favorite student during the preparation exercises, in an effort to harden herself to the worst possible eventuality." A Faster instructor was quite encouraging of such resolve: "If we can have them win in their minds first, against that student, then when it comes to the actual incident they will prevail."[14]

What an astounding proposition, this tragic lesson about winning "in their minds first, against that student." This adherence to a toxic shoot-'em-up Wild West ethic puts teachers in a clear bind: they must labor from the untenable position of actively imagining their students in the crosshairs, the objects of target practice.

Deputizing teachers as locked-and-loaded "peace" officers speaks volumes about how challenged police are by the quotidian nature of gun violence. It should make us ponder how democratic assumptions about the state having a monopoly on violence have been frayed by anarchic ideologies of "every man for himself." It brings that us-versus-them mentality into the classroom. The Colorado teacher imagined her favorite student; I'm guessing that many would imagine their worst student, or some stereotype of dangerous otherness. Either way, the imaginative act of seeing the best as worst and the worst as expendable is a separate danger in itself—a premeditated license to shoot faster, ever faster.

In the United States, more than half the population believes that having a gun enhances the chances of survival in a world overrun by gangs of terrorists, but the data show very conclusively that gun ownership is much more likely to *increase* the risk of harm. Research shows, as *Slate* notes, "a gun in the home was far more likely to be used to threaten a family member or intimate partner than to be used in self-defense." According to the Brady Campaign to Prevent Gun Violence, not only is "the risk of homicide . . . three times higher in homes with firearms," but in addition, "keeping a firearm in the home increases the risk of suicide by a factor of 3 to 5 and increases the risk of suicide with a firearm by a factor of 17."[15] There is no reason to suppose that such figures wouldn't apply to gun-centered classrooms. It's hard to comprehend this foolish disregard of empirical data about what actually reduces gun violence.

When the nuclear-warning system accidentally went off in Hawaii a few years ago, many experienced the profound helplessness of confronting an unfathomable force of violence. Perhaps it lends a certain sense of control to imagine that we'd have time to "protect" ourselves by crawling into an air-raid shelter, but in a real nuclear attack, anyone within a broad range would be incinerated instantly. The only real hope for survival would have been limiting and controlling the weapons themselves.

The same holds true for the extraordinary arsenal that Americans own privately. We can do our best to protect ourselves against every unexpected irrational attack like the one in Las Vegas in 2017, which killed 60 people and wounded 413.[16] But unless we wrap our bodies perpetually in Kevlar and travel in bomb-resistant tanks, the problem remains: too many guns are in circulation. It is foolish to imagine that we might protect ourselves without reducing the number. In America, guns exact a toll greater than that of active warfare. According to *The Guardian*, between 1968 and 2015,

> there have been 1,516,863 gun-related deaths on US territory. Since the founding of the United States, there have been 1,396,733 war deaths. That figure includes American lives lost in the Revolutionary War, the Mexican War, the Civil War (Union and Confederate), the Spanish-American War, the First World War, the Second World War, the Korean War, the Vietnam War, the Gulf War, the Afghanistan War, the Iraq War, as well as other conflicts, including in Lebanon, Grenada, Panama, Somalia, and Haiti.[17]

As if that weren't bad enough, between 2019 and 2020, the firearm homicide rate in America increased by a stunning 35 percent.[18] As I write this sentence in the unfinished year 2023, there have been more mass shootings in the United States than days in the year.

Sometimes I wake up with a strange recurring dream, captioned in neon, no less, as "The New State of Equality." In it, every American has a gun pointed at the person in front of them or the person behind them. If anyone starts shooting, everyone dies in the chaos that inevitably ensues. I mentioned this disruptive nightmare to a colleague, describing it as my clearly defined sense of a fuse about to be lit. My colleague saw it differently: such a conceptual standoff is a good thing to him. No one dares make a sudden move, he maintains. He thinks this is precisely the appropriate balance for civil society: everyone must be really careful and "make nice."

Against a backdrop of such ubiquitous trauma, I suppose the Buckeye Foundation's Faster training for teachers maps rather neatly onto an American romance with redemptive vigilantism. I use the word "romance" advisedly—for all the risks of gun possession, there is something gleeful, almost celebratory in the posturing of the most ardent defenders of the Second Amendment, like Representatives Thomas Massie and Lauren Boebert. It reminds me of Jean-Paul Sartre's short story "Erostratus," in which the narrator derives misanthropic and sexual pleasure from carrying a gun hidden in his pocket. That exhilaration comes, he says, not from the gun, but rather "from myself: I was a being like a revolver, a torpedo, or a bomb." Philosopher Roberto Esposito writes that "things constitute the filter through which humans . . . enter into relationship with each other." Guns, torpedoes, and bombs are precisely such things. Warns Esposito: "The more our technological objects, with the know-how that has made them serviceable, embody a sort of subjective life, the less we can squash them into an exclusively servile function."[19]

7
Erasure

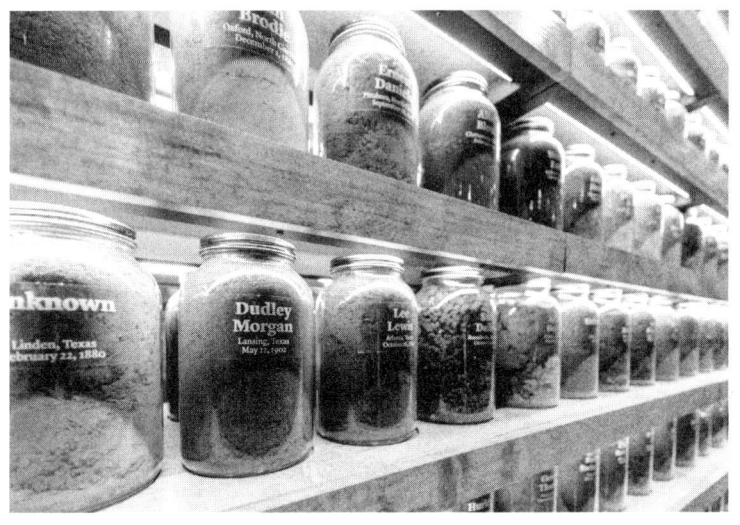

Hundreds of jars of soil from documented lynching sites, featured at the Legacy Museum as part of the National Memorial for Peace and Justice in Montgomery, Alabama[1]

Audra Melton/*The New York Times*/Redux

If anyone wonders about the enduringly violent trauma in which America so persistently finds itself awash, it is certainly worth studying the pattern of extrajudicial killings that slavery licensed but that continued with increased and unremediated fervor in the wake of Reconstruction through the Jim Crow era. I have become particularly interested in this period because of the scholarship of Professor Margaret A. Burnham, the founding director of Northeastern University's

Civil Rights and Restorative Justice Project, which has spent close to two decades excavating more than a thousand unresolved cases of racially motivated beatings, kidnappings, disappearances, and deaths between 1920 and 1960. It is impossible to read about this body of cases without noting the chilling similarity to the string of unremediated cases that plague us today, which are the subject of so much contemporary organizing, including the Black Lives Matter movement.

"If the law cannot protect a person from a lynching, then isn't lynching the law?" This question frames the CRRJ project's investigations and is explored in Burnham's book about the project, *By Hands Now Known: Jim Crow's Legal Executioners*.[2] Along with digital archivist Melissa Nobles, professor of political science at MIT, Burnham enlisted teams of researchers, local officials, students, cartographers, journalists, and living witnesses, as well as hundreds of family members and far-flung descendants of both victims and perpetrators. They combed through newspaper accounts, coroners' reports, photo albums, church records, legal briefs, and graveyards. The sum of those tens of thousands of hours of labor is accessible online at the Burnham-Nobles Digital Archive, crrjarchive.org. Besides the remarkable data collected in the digital archive, the book brings lost lives to life in a way that ties private family histories to the wider public story of lethal state violence, as evidenced not only in extrajudicial killings but also by the widespread failure to prosecute anyone at all for so many murders of Black citizenry. "It was our sense," writes Burnham, "that as long as these events translated as idiosyncratic, one-off, private experiences of grief, multifaceted systems of racial injustice would remain hidden, and concomitantly, the need for structural remedies would seem unwarranted."[3]

There were several common arenas of legal failure. First was the practice of rendition using the Fugitive Felon Act, which allowed Southern lawmen to travel across state lines with warrants demanding the return of Blacks who had fled to the North to avoid lynch mobs.

Second was the dangerous geography of public transportation. Gun-toting bus drivers were the chief enforcers of Jim Crow laws determining the size of Colored Only sections, adjusting the number of rows and answering to white patrons whose desire for more seating was determinative. Bus drivers could push Black patrons off buses for any or no reason. They could and did kill Blacks for back talk or bad attitude. Third, there was (then as now) the systemic practice of immunizing state actors like police officers, so that even the most brutal misdeeds went unprosecuted and unpunished. Fourth, the federal government—including the federal bench and the Supreme Court—utterly abandoned its duty to enforce those provisions of Reconstruction-era laws that prohibited states' allowance of racist terror.

The era of terror known as the Redemption (of Confederate interests) was occasioned not only by the withdrawal of federal troops in the wake of the Hayes-Tilden Compromise of 1877, but also by the judiciary's introducing a notion of dual federalism that ceded primary enforcement of civil rights to states rather than to the federal government. This instantiation of "states' rights" was the portal to the lethal logics of Jim Crow's ideology of "separate but equal." Thus, the brief hope of Reconstruction's assurances to the formerly enslaved pretty much ended with the 1876 case of *United States v. Cruikshank*, which concluded that victims of civil and political rights violations should "look to the states" for primary recourse.[4] As Burnham observes, Black people "had to depend on their former owners to protect their newly gained federal rights."[5]

Later decisions, like *Screws v. United States* in 1945, introduced an even higher bar for federal intervention, by introducing a novel and virtually unprovable element of "willful" intent that federal prosecutors had to show in bringing indictments for murderous civil rights violations.[6] Georgia sheriff Claude Screws harbored a self-proclaimed grudge against one Robert Hall, a young Black man whom he arrested, handcuffed, and then beat to death with his fists and a two-pound metal blackjack. An indictment was procured under Section 52 of the Federal Penal Code, which makes it a crime for a public official intentionally to violate an individual's constitutional rights. However, despite evidence that Sheriff Screws had announced in advance that he planned to "get the Black SOB and . . . kill him" because he had "lived too long,"[7] the Supreme Court overturned the indictment, writing that, while the law was indeed an "anti-discrimination law . . . framed to protect Negroes in their newly won rights," federal prosecution thereunder demanded proof that "the accused had the willful intent to violate a right of the victim that was specifically guaranteed by the Constitution . . . in this case the right to a regular judicial proceeding, rather than, as Justice Douglas put it, 'trial by ordeal.'"[8] The impossible burden of proving willful intent to transgress a specific constitutional provision doomed the project of federal civil rights enforcement for decades more, and the insistent segregationist assertion of states' rights allowed "authoritarian southern political systems [to thrive] within an ostensibly democratic national polity."[9]

The sheer number of cases unearthed by the Civil Rights and Restorative Justice Project makes clear that the deployment of threats and violence were systemic features of Jim Crow, part of a regime that carried forward slavery's cruelest assumptions—not only that Blacks could not testify against whites, but that the killing of a Black person by a white person was a mostly private matter, a presumptive "accident" of the anti-insurrectionist discipline necessary to preserve the intimacies of social order. This logic was sustained by habitual denial of access to the public infrastructure of law enforcement: outright murder was simultaneously condoned and ignored by police, politicians, media, coroners, and the judicial system. Shrouding violence behind disclaimers of Southern chivalry and "honor preserved" thus became a practice of hiding profound acts of brutality.

It is worth hovering over this point, for we live in a moment when revived claims that slavery was benevolent and that segregation reflected mere social preference seem to be reshaping how history will be taught—or whether it will be taught at all. A wide range of politicians—from former President Trump to governors including Florida's Ron DeSantis, Texas's Greg Abbott, and Virginia's Glenn Youngkin—have staked their reputations upon how quickly they can erase from public libraries and school curricula any information that is potentially "upsetting" or "uncomfortable" or "distressing." Indeed, the anti–critical race theory laws that have been enacted in more than thirty states as of this writing do not seem to have any coherent definition of what they are outlawing, but they are very clear in their rejection of the notion that racism could possibly be systemic, or widespread, or officially encouraged, or historically important. Margaret Burnham's account in *By Hands Now Known* profoundly challenges the denialism that says slavery's violent aftereffects in America are "exceptional" or occasional. Indeed, for at least the last two centuries, American jurisprudence of civil rights has been explicitly entangled with—and tangled up by—legally inscribed hierarchies of racism's sorrows and exclusions, enduring to the present. Burnham identifies direct physical violence as a "defining feature of Jim Crow . . . transforming, in fundamental ways, concepts of federalism, citizenship, and democratic rights and privileges."[10]

Thus, *By Hands Now Known* must not be read as though it were a laundry list of singular case after singular case. The reiterated frequency of violent death reveals regional and collective practices, patterns, and cultures, with repeated offenses and repeat offenders. The atmospheric trauma of such crimes enforced "a form of sub-citizenship" that did not just weigh on emotional life, but frustrated the ability to protest, to appeal, or to mourn.[11] Victims lost their lives, and that loss was repercussive: families lost fathers, mothers, children, jobs, homes, farms, businesses, and hope. Black people fled the Deep South in such droves that the entire landscape of the United States was transformed.

Jim Crow's violence and the impoverishing conditions of servitude were primary causes of the Great Migration, lasting from 1910 until about 1970. As Isabel Wilkerson documents in her book *The Warmth of Other Suns*, that exodus of more than 6 million Black people from the rural South to the urban North remains one of the largest internal migrations in human history.[12]

The notion that such massive and desperate fleeing was *not* a response to systemic racial tribulation speaks also to the systemic nature of enforced oblivion. In addition to physical separation, the laws of segregation imposed separate worlds of memory. In interviews with the families of white perpetrators, the CRRJ team encountered children and grandchildren who had been told stories of heroic intervention, such as "He was running at me. I had to shoot!" When confronted with something like a coroner's report showing that the victim was instead shot repeatedly in the back, responses ranged from confusion and disbelief to deep distress, as the narrative structure of gilded family innocence cracked and fell apart. In interviews with the families of Black victims, on the other hand, descendants are more likely to respond with relief at finally being able to talk about it—as in, "This explains a lot about my grandmother's terrible sadness!"

The agents of extralegal execution, whether police or private citizens, also had the power to isolate and control Black resistance—even to prevent Black people from just talking about it among themselves, as in church services or at funerals. This control was magnified by active erasures of the terror—by hiding bodies in graves with no markers, by dumping the dead in rivers or otherwise "losing" bodies, by destroying evidence, or simply by deciding to omit such murders from newspapers or other historical accounts. These acts of suppression were woven into walls of silence, so that even the most horrendously traumatic crimes might go not merely unpunished but unpublished as well, the stories rendered invisible and all inquiry taboo. Black lives melted quickly from collective memory, unable to be spoken of or acknowledged, though they might be held silently in the muffled hearts of widows and orphans. While the African American press and the NAACP did their best to track injustices, an epistemic crisis of "not knowing" took hold on diverse planes of culture—lost to forensic or actuarial account, lost from the responsibilities of political address.

In unearthing the mundanity of violence during Jim Crow, one can trace the links between antebellum slave-catching laws and policing practices that have lasted to this day. Indeed, it is hard *not* to see parallels between the Fugitive Slave Act's "commissioning" of white citizens to find and return "larcenous" runaways (the larceny being the paradoxical theft of "their own" yet "not their own" bodies) and today's broadly delegated enforcement of antiabortion laws, like Texas's SB8, which would pay private persons, neighbors, and random strangers to hunt down and retrieve for prosecution any women who might think of having an abortion.

The exuberant prevalence of civilians arresting civilians without warrant has a particular history in the American context. Its seemingly unbounded popularity and its deployment even today are a direct legacy of laws that paid private citizens a bounty to hunt down Blacks trying to escape slavery or oppressive contract labor. As a circuit court judge justified the kidnapping and false imprisonment of a Black man in 1946: "The right of private arrest is just as sacred and just as important to the public interest as that of arrest by an officer armed with a warrant."[13]

The not-knowing of so many deaths is worthy of its own unpacking. The Civil Rights and Restorative Justice Project revelations are not limited to the law's failing to investigate or refusing to prosecute. Most important, these cases also show a pattern of censorship and a steep price for speaking truth—although the truth was often winkingly revealed in clearly fudged police reports, newspaper articles, death certificates, or coroners' reports. Any public criticism or calling to account was habitually met with retribution. To be sure, there was a lot of not-caring in the un-documentary practice that repeatedly inscribed "unknown" upon so many official forms. But those gaps and omissions may be read as well, perhaps, as the collectively powerful conformities of fear. So, while this accumulated history is surely difficult and disquieting for its own sake, it is also a history of crimes whose murkiness rests upon the powerful architecture of *public secrets*. As anthropologist Michael Taussig has written, public secrets retain an almost religious power because their often murderous agents extract retribution upon revelation or complaint.[14] Public secrets rely on whole societies' knowing what not to know.

Toni Morrison wrote of the "nightmare" world of lost voices where it is "as though a whole universe is being written in invisible ink." She observed, "Certain kinds of trauma visited on peoples are so deep, so cruel, that unlike money, unlike vengeance, even unlike justice, or rights, or the goodwill of others, only writers can translate such trauma and turn sorrow into meaning, sharpening the moral imagination.... A writer's life and work are not a gift to mankind, they are its necessity."[15]

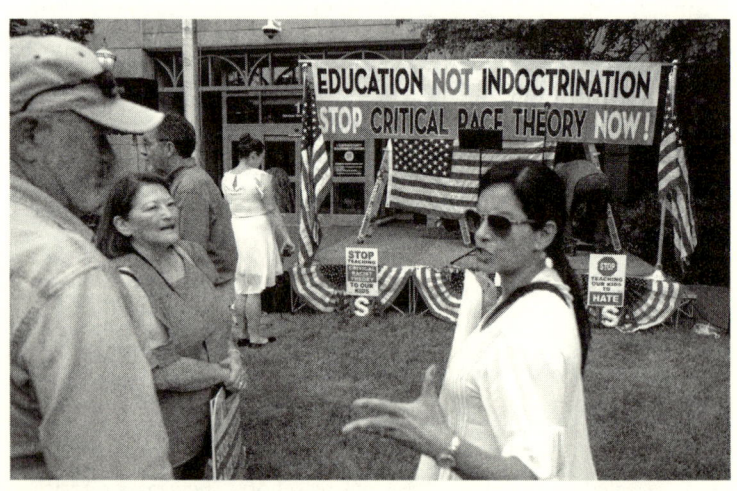

Theory conspiracy: A rally protesting the teaching of critical race theory at the Loudoun County Government Center in Leesburg, Virginia

Andrew Caballero-Reynolds/AFP

That said, it is ironic that Margaret Burnham's careful resurrection of what was obliterated but is "now known" was published at the precise moment when political forces in the United States began rapidly organizing to push those histories right back into the closet, with a flotilla of Make-Sure-You-Don't-Know laws that radically proscribe the ability of students of all ages to learn or read about uncomfortable aspects of our history. The work of the Civil Rights and Restorative Justice Project leaves us to wonder: Given a legacy of such horror that even "to mourn was to dissent" because "to mourn was to defy what law wrought,"[16] how can a case for justice be crafted that might resist lies, denialism, and retributive propaganda? That irony seems particularly important to bear in mind amid today's political maelstrom, where some politicians demonize teachers, librarians, books, Black people, gay people, undecided people, trans people, liberal people, and even Mickey Mouse; and when teachers, librarians, administrators, and whole school districts are losing their jobs, losing funding—punished for discussing Black politics and history and what has been done to Black as well as queer bodies.

Enforced silence is an important feature of Jim Crow's legacy of racial retribution. Current book banning, one must not forget, is part of a longer history of anti-literacy campaigns targeting Black and other minority expression. During slavery it was a punishable offense to teach Blacks to read or write, or even to allow them to work at a printing press. After Emancipation, the Black Codes of the late 1800s suppressed Black self-expression including writing or publishing, discouraged education, forbade voting, penalized attempts to assemble, and outlawed Blacks from testifying against whites in court. Indeed, four years before her printing press was destroyed for publishing lynching statistics, Ida B. Wells-Barnett was fired from her job as a teacher in the Memphis public schools because she complained publicly about the dismally degrading conditions of the few segregated Black schools that existed.[17]

I am among the first generation of "affirmative action babies," whose sudden visible numbers offended many people by our very presence. We brought with us family histories that were entangled with and embarrassed the Founding Fathers—from Thomas Jefferson to Strom Thurmond. We challenged notions that enslaved underaged women might have consensually engaged in "love affairs" with their married masters. We posited reinterpretations that completed histories, contradicted comfortable assumptions, talked, and talked back. Often inadvertently, we opened those prohibited cans of worms still writhing in the American underbelly; we complicated the history to which so many forgetful Americans yearn to return "again."

The shared longing for a sunnier future sometimes seems to be twisted into nostalgia for a fictitious sunnier past: an implicit instruction to shut up about the past and just assimilate already. It's hard, even for a very privileged Black person, to "assimilate" into a world featuring so many elephants in every room, and with so many people taught to act as though they're not there. An African American friend describes a familiar scenario: "My son L. was invited to a neighbor's seventh birthday party. When we arrived, the neighbor child introduced L. to the small circle of other children, all of whom were white; he did so in hushed tones, seemingly so that adults wouldn't hear. 'This is my friend L.,' he whispered. 'He's Black!' He said it with giddy pride, as though L. were an exotic prize, an unusual triumph, a trophy specimen."

What struck my friend most was not that the children were marveling at Blackness as something they had seemingly never encountered, but that the young host whispered it. "He was self-conscious," she said. "He lowered his voice as though he had learned that he shouldn't say it aloud, that it was a kind of secret—if in plain sight." He had somehow learned that race shouldn't be seen, and that the conspicuity of Blackness imposed a burden of comportment.

My friend was pulled up short by it at the time, but after thought and discussion about what she might do in the future, she concluded that the situation required something simple, like an adult in the room who might have calmly intervened and told them that they didn't have to whisper. Why were they acting as though it were a secret? The tougher question, of course, is for the other adults: Why might this have been the first time their children had seen a Black person? Children point at, whisper about, marvel at what they don't know. But the reason for an integrated education is to get to know one another in generally welcoming ways.

Here's my grown-up tug of recognition about that birthday party: I graduated from law school in 1975. The movie *The Paper Chase* came out around that time, and if you've ever seen it, you've seen law school as it was when I attended Harvard: almost entirely white, almost entirely male. No tenure-track women on the faculty and only one recently hired Black man, Derrick Bell. Those numbers alone could account for why Professor Bell is often hailed as the founder of critical race theory: at the very least he was a portal to Black lawyers thinking aloud. Indeed, the very fact of minorities and women appearing in that space at that time often marked us as contrarian upstarts before we even opened our mouths. Our numbers would change for the better (if not by much) thanks to affirmative action (despite much rhetoric about minorities "taking over"), but even such relatively small gains in previously homogeneous cartographies make some people feel as though they are drowning among the unfamiliar and the undeserving.

Students in those days learned about the "reasonable man" standard in criminal law, under which the murder of one's wandering wife could be mitigated by the "heat of passion" defense. In constitutional law, I learned everything there was to know about the commerce clause, but nary a word about the civil rights struggle to overturn Jim Crow laws and integrate workplaces, unions, schools, bathrooms, neighborhoods. That "extra" material was confined to optional elective classes. The few classes about minority interests were sifted out and segregated from the required courses.

When I started teaching in 1980, I was one of eight women of color teaching law in the entire United States, including at historically Black colleges: six African Americans, one Asian American, and one Latina. In those early years, men in my various workplaces openly and routinely commented on my hair, clothes, weight, legs, waist, age, skin color, voice, accent, makeup or lack thereof, jewelry (no ring?!), and marital status. My body felt spitted and twirled over a fire of others' curiosity.

Make no mistake, I understand being curious about what one has never seen. Humans settle into perceived orders, and as those orders shift, people who appear "out of place" may find themselves marked, remarked on, exoticized, or shunned. But those experiences made me think deeply about how to be a thoughtful adult in the room of that curiosity. How do we move past the surrealism of "alien" encounters and begin to address the social uneasiness festering from invisible history, bad manners, mutual ignorance, and unfettered in-your-face curiosity?

The very presence of new faces during those early years of my career forged new connections, new ways of thinking. We began to speak across all kinds of boundaries: disciplinary, linguistic, ontological—what Professor Kimberlé Crenshaw (founder of the African American Policy Forum) later called "intersectional" work.

Professor Bell was a kind, thoughtful man, and thus an important progenitor of such conversation. He worked tirelessly to recenter dropped histories. He'd point out how disabling racially restrictive covenants were, not just as a topic for a separate course on "race law" but as integral to the power relations within foundational courses like property law. He invited everyone of that generation into an open circle of knowledge-seeking about how to deal with varied alignments of social power. The early writers in this genre included professors

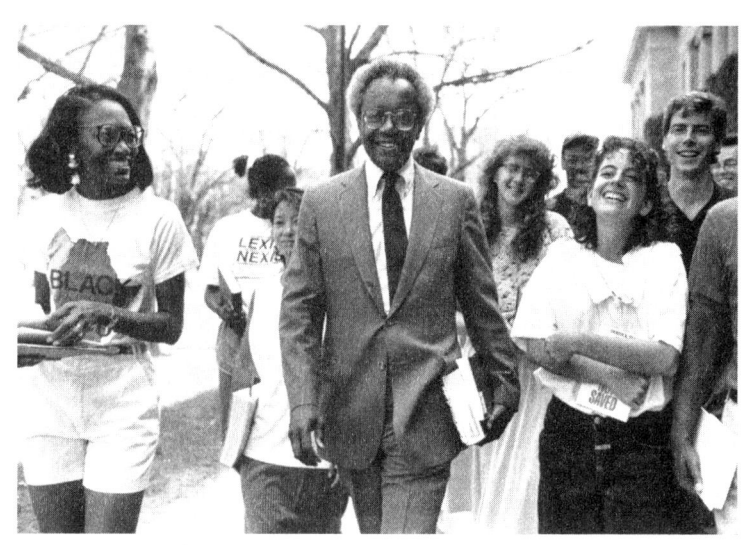

Steve Liss/Getty Images[18]

Charles Lawrence, Mari Matsuda, Gary Peller, Gerald Torres, Paulette Caldwell, Robert Williams, Dorothy Roberts, Regina Austin, Eric Yamamoto, Harlon Dalton, Jerome Culp, Richard Delgado, Jean Stefancic, Kendall Thomas, Cheryl Harris, Kimberlé Crenshaw, and an interdisciplinary handful of others.

The body of writing that emerged referenced a broad range of interdisciplinary scholarly movements, engaging with the insights of legal realism and feminist jurisprudence, as well as with figures from the still-new critical legal studies movement, such as Duncan Kennedy, Roberto Unger, Morton Horwitz, and Peter Gabel. Those diversely integrative connections were the origins of critical race theory—although I have always thought of what Bell started as a "critical race conversation" rather than a theory. It is out of this era's grappling with the history and experience of legalized marginalization that critical race theory was born. The era marked the simultaneous emergence of critical feminist theory, of "Latcrit" (scholarship about Latin and Hispanic identities), of revisitations of indigenous rights and treaties, of discussions about the status of migrant workers, and of conversations about the jurisprudence of gay rights. It was a time of great transformation; it was a productive time, a hopeful, even a joyful time.

The work begun then is still reverberating, still unfolding. But social change, particularly in the domain of race, has never gone unchallenged. If we are in a moment where such resistance is suddenly greater than in the recent past, there's still a familiar shape to the aversion.

Here's a story from 2021 about what happens when anxiously whispering children grow up: In Traverse City, Michigan, a community more than 90 percent white, a group of high school students formed a Snapchat group called "Slave Trade," in which they ruminated that "all Blacks should die" and suggested "let's start another holocaust."[19] The contents of their online exchanges became public only after they'd held a slave auction, selling off their Black classmates for money. "I know how much I was sold for: $100," said one girl who was "traded" thus. "And in the end I was given away for free."[20]

When all this came to light, the school quickly drafted a resolution to create a social equity task force committed to "recognizing that the actions needed to combat discrimination and racism depend on new knowledge and community progress." But the draft resolution became the object of fierce resistance from some parents, who, as of this writing, have succeeded in editing out language encouraging a "social equity and diversity lens" for the curriculum; taking out a promise to add books by "marginalized" authors to school libraries; cutting mention of teaching about "diversity, equity, inclusion and belonging issues"; removing language condemning "racism," "racial violence," "hate speech," and "bigotry"; and removing the statement "racism and hate have no place in our schools or in our society." The largely parent-driven backlash has led to the excising of the very vocabulary that would enable speakers of the English language to say that slave-trading one's Black classmates on Snapchat is wrong.[21]

This story illustrates all the unfortunate dynamics of how *not* to talk about race—indeed, how not to talk about anything at all. It demonstrates the degree to which some parents view race like sex: taboo, prurient, something to keep hidden because it'll give the children fevers and make the parents squirm. As with sex, ignorance about race becomes a secret excitement; racial disparagement becomes an indulgent exercise, a species of cathartic emphasis, like swear words. For many children who are socialized as not-different, and for the normatively comfortable adults they become, discussion of race remains stunted and infantile, too much like assigning "cooties"—loosely undefined yet cruelly specific. So you ban sex education in the name of chastity, purity, innocence. You ban talk about race that is inherently "divisive." But when Americans of different races greet each other as though they had just stepped off a ship in 1492, let's just say that the division is glaringly already there. It begs to be addressed.

At the school board meetings in Traverse City, the very notion of an equity resolution was, as one parent put it, "interlaced with critical race theory." Parents held signs and testified that they considered the resolution "Marxist," "anti-Christian," "divisive," and "anti-white." I have read the resolution in both its original and edited form; there is nothing in either that hints of Marxism or of the Antichrist.[22] Indeed, it's quite a mystery why fear of the "divisive" would require eliminating antonyms like "inclusion and belonging." It is a sign of the confusion of this moment that condemning racist language or bullying behavior is seen as the automatic and specific equivalent of being "anti-white."

At the public hearings, most parents seemed to minimize the fact that many of their kids—many more, by all accounts, than an isolated Snapchat group—saw fit to disparage, humiliate, dehumanize, and even call for the killing of their nonwhite classmates. Instead, the greater sin, according to the parental pushback, was that "race" was ever mentioned at all. Darcie Pickren, one of the most-quoted parent leaders, maintained: "We don't, not even for a second, think about race. We never would. And I think that this is opening a can of worms and we are not going to be able to go back." Pickren feared that "schools have been revising their curriculums . . . and basically saying we're going to cancel math and English to bring in these social justice studies instead." To Pickren, teaching social justice studies "sounds like we're going to be teaching our kids our country is founded on racism and show them that if they're white, they're privileged and they're part of the problem."[23]

Since 2020, an alternative, ugly, defamatory, made-up impersonation of critical race theory has muscled aside the actual history and now dominates a reign of malignant confusion, targeting and tarring gay people, trans people, immigrants, Jews, Muslims, Asians, women, pregnancy, contraception, and whole realms of science. This remarkable season of backlash began in earnest in early 2020, with racialized attacks on writings about very particular aspects of Black history, the Black Lives Matter movement, and conversations about racial repair. The attacks were focused particularly against works that foregrounded enslavement in the context of America's origin story, such as the *New York Times* 1619 Project, or those that have encouraged conversations about repair—including the freighted topic of reparations, such as Ta-Nahisi Coates's *Between the World and Me*.[24]

These attacks were neither random nor grassroots; they were engineered and stoked by a very careful and cynical propaganda campaign. While the culture wars have plagued us for the past thirty years, the peculiar bitterness of this iteration began only in September 2020, with former president Donald Trump's now rescinded executive order banning critical race theory and diversity training in all federal programs. It's worth looking back at the language of that order, which was jaw-dropping in its specious linkage of critical race theory to both hate and contagion. As Trump wrote in a follow-up tweet: "This is a sickness that cannot be allowed to continue. Please report any sightings so we can quickly extinguish!"[25]

"Extinguish," no less! This is a sentiment that far exceeds concern about either history or bad pedagogy. It evacuates the meaning of critical race theory as an academic discussion, one that began decades ago in law schools. This definitional theft treats the mere discussion of race as a disease and a poison. It lifts the topic of race from the contentious to the deadly; it deploys an executive order to authorize censorship; it carries the imperative of a search-and-destroy surveillance mission with the express goal of quick extinction.

Christopher Rufo, a senior analyst at the Manhattan Institute, is widely credited with being the ideological picador behind Trump's 2020 executive order. He dragged the little-known concept from its narrow jurisprudential corner and wholly redefined it—and did so in utter bad faith. In a much-cited Twitter thread just after the executive order was issued, Rufo stated that his goal was to "run a public persuasion campaign" that would conflate any number of topics and deposit them into a new bucket called critical race theory. "We have successfully frozen their brand—'critical race theory'—into the public conversation and are steadily driving up negative perceptions," he wrote. "We will eventually turn it toxic, as we put all of the various cultural insanities under that brand category. . . . The goal is to have the public read something crazy in the newspaper and immediately think 'critical race theory.' We have decodified the term and will recodify it to annex the entire range of cultural constructions that are unpopular with Americans."[26]

And so he has—or so the mysterious "we" have. Within a year, almost every Republican candidate in the country had sworn to eliminate the evil entity passing as "critical race theory."

By 2023, Rufo had become Florida governor Ron DeSantis's favored picador, invited to help with state and local enforcement of Florida's so-called Stop WOKE Act. He remains straightforward about his political ends: "I basically took that body of criticism, I paired it with breaking news stories that were shocking and explicit and horrifying, and made it political," he said. "Turned it into a salient political issue with a clear villain."[27]

This is what "critical race theory" has become: an effigy. It is whatever the world-creating powers of Rufo or Tucker Carlson or the Conservative Political Action Coalition or QAnon says it is. It is a million imaginary Black drag queens dressed up as teachers hired to feast on the brains of kindergartners, killing their innocence. It is a term reduced to a floating signifier, never defined—a child-snatching, innocence-killing, academic Willie Horton of a concept.

By 2022, CRT, as it was reductively known by then, had indeed been "recodified," *in actual law* no less, as anything that made people feel guilty, shamed, or blamed. Frighteningly, former president Donald Trump has used it in attempts to motivate actual violence, literally calling for sacrifice at a rally in South Carolina: "Getting critical race theory out of our schools is not just a matter of values, it's also a matter of national survival. We have no choice. The fate of any nation ultimately depends upon the willingness of its citizens to lay down—and they must do this—lay down their very lives to defend their country."[28]

What clearer proof can there be of our so easily reactivated historical traumas? "The task of propaganda," wrote Joseph Goebbels, "is not to say as much as possible, but rather to gather completely confused, complex, and composite ideas into a single catch phase and then to instill this into the people as a whole."[29]

Although Trump's 2020 executive order was revoked by President Biden, Republicans have since crafted nearly identical prohibitions against teaching true history in public schools or employee training, and have introduced such bills in state legislatures with lightning rapidity. These laws have been enacted in whole or in part in at least thirty-six states. As of 2022, just before the midterm elections, only eight states have not seen anti-CRT bills introduced. Republicans have announced their intention to federalize a version of anti-CRT and anti-LGBTQ laws if they can take control of Congress in 2024.

In the maelstrom of such rapidly coordinated political backlash, school boards around the country have exploded in painful, community-destroying bouts of antagonism. The language of the laws is almost identical, having been drafted not at the local level but by a team coordinated and funded by an array of conservative think tanks, including the Manhattan Institute, the American Enterprise Institute, and the Heritage Foundation. That template starts off seemingly innocently by mandating that there shall be no stereotyping by race or sex; no instruction that teaches that any one race or sex is inherently superior to another; no teaching that any individual is intrinsically racist, sexist, or oppressive; and no teaching that anyone bears automatic responsibility for actions committed in the past by members of the same race. So far, so good. But in a perverse twist, the bills characterize these noble ideas as *anti*–critical race theory. By this illogic, such laws strongly—and wrongly—imply that critical race theory advocates all the crude biological determinism that the laws ban.

And the bills and laws go further. Most bar "mandatory gender or sexual diversity training" and discussion of "controversial" topics; some ban teaching the 1619 Project. Others, like Alabama's, propose to ban critical race theory "outright"—and then define it as any belief that America is inherently racist or sexist, "whether consciously or unconsciously." Nearly all versions prohibit teaching in which "any individual should feel discomfort, guilt, anguish or any other form of psychological distress on account of his or her race or sex."

This last is perhaps the most troubling of all the provisions: The discomfort of public school students—from kindergarten through college—becomes, per se, a violation that may invoke monetary fines for teachers, risk their being fired, or result in withholding funds from individual schools or whole districts. In effect, the emotions of young children and immature youth become a metric for disciplining teachers and educational institutions. If students become upset about difficult dialogues, heads will roll.

The sudden proliferation of identically worded laws not only suppresses conversation about race in schools and workplaces but also "deputizes" citizen spies. (The Nevada Family Alliance, an advocacy group, has even urged that teachers be forced to wear body cameras, like police officers, to make sure that they aren't "indoctrinating" students to "hate America.") This deputizing of citizens is in keeping with the new abortion law in Texas that incentivizes citizens to inform on each other, and those that allow patrols of armed poll watchers in open-carry states.

This framing makes it impossible to do what I am too often requested to do—to tell you what critical race theory is—for this is no longer a definitional or a factual dispute. Like all good propaganda, its object exists in the bleary eye of the beholder. Critical race theory has been positioned as th.at which cannot be defined because Rufo et al. have transformed it from an epistemic referent into an emotional repository. It is well-spun sorcery, a haze of hate. It is a gestural assignment of social contagion that operates like magic.

What is especially pernicious about these new bills and laws is that they outlaw feelings, which transfers agency beyond negotiation or norm. They remove the power of conformity with the law from the intentions of teachers and displace that power onto the emotions of children. Fox News touts stories of mixed-up mixed-race children who come home from school claiming to have been taught that their white daddy is the mean oppressor of their Asian/Latina/African

American mommy. I'm sure that there are teachers who get things disastrously wrong, but honestly, it takes something less than a law to untangle that one—and less than a civil war. We have gotten our wires seriously crossed. Teaching hard histories to children really is simpler than a national emergency.

In a world of good faith, we work hard to bridge the distances between us. Skilled role models can teach us how not to shame and humiliate one another; it takes commitment to press through the freighted emotions that any controversial subject might evoke. I believe in teaching teachers how to broach difficult subjects—"diversity training," for lack of a better term. Such teaching must include not only historical fact but analytical thought, methodologies of discernment, diplomacy, patience, listening skills, and creating enough trust to cry, get angry, and forgive.

Any law that bans specific books, pieces of journalism, or words from generalized classroom discussion is galloping down a path of reductive fundamentalism or authoritarianism. This is not to say that there shouldn't be disciplinary processes to hear arguments about what constitutes a hostile learning or work environment, or what ought to be disciplined as un-collegial or anti-intellectual behavior. Unlike outright bans on speech, however, the disciplinary procedures already present in our jurisprudence judge the propriety of what is taught by putting individual cases and controversies in context. It's what human resources departments negotiate, or tenure reviews investigate, or harassment rules hash out. In contrast, the new anti–critical race theory laws ban whole categories of speech not yet spoken.

Ten years ago, absolutist "free speech" bullies like Rush Limbaugh fought endlessly to say whatever they damn well pleased, loudly and on the public airwaves. Now some of the very same blowhards are bullying legislatively to prevent words or concepts from being spoken or taught. (Their efforts have flattened meanings past the point of mere irony, all the way to absurdity: even as I wrote "damn well pleased," the autocorrect function on my computer popped up to warn me, "This language may be offensive to your reader.") At either extreme, it's the same dangerous paradox: the manipulation of who can speak with unfettered impunity and who cannot.

We cannot legislate feelings about race into silence. Outlawing shame, guilt, and discomfort is not only silly and impossible, but it also positions race the same way blasphemy laws position speaking ill of God or the king. Looking at the difficult parts of our lives as Americans is not sacrilege; we do not (yet) live in a sacred order whose holiness is sullied by impingements of the impure.

Alas, ridiculous extremes have spread like herpes. Recently an angry man sent bomb threats to Merriam-Webster's headquarters because he disagreed with the company's dictionaries' definition of *woman*, *girl*, and *female*. "There is no such thing as gender identity," he proclaimed.[30] A friend tells me that a child in her son's kindergarten got upset because a poster of the first Thanksgiving included "people who aren't white"—he meant American Indians—"and that's against the law." Imagine how much noisily shushing nonsense that small child had digested, to think any inclusion of brown faces is a racial wrong.

Of course, all this raises the question of what happens if the adults truly don't know. A British friend tells me about a generally well-educated American woman who was completing her doctorate in the UK. During a class, someone asked her about the American Civil War. The young American had no idea what they were talking about. It took some explanation before she realized they were talking about what she knew only as "the war of Northern aggression." It is sometimes startling how bunkered we are, how already divided we are and have been.

Recently a historian friend sent me a snippet from the 2012 platform from the Texas Republican Party convention: "Knowledge-Based Education—We oppose the teaching of Higher Order Thinking Skills (values clarification), critical thinking skills, and similar programs that are simply a relabeling of Outcome-based Education (mastery learning) which focus on behavior modification and have the purpose of challenging the students' fixed beliefs and undermining parental authority." This was eye-opening. It made me realize the degree to which race is not our only divide. This provision was widely derided and mocked as extreme when it was added to the convention platform back in 2012. All it took was Christopher Rufo's adding the ingredient of race—"critical thinking skills" became relabeled "critical race skills"—to popularize it as an instant Republican bogeyman.

This Republican platform plank also made me aware that to some Americans, teaching is not really about encouraging students to think critically about anything, including race. For them, teaching is not about challenging students to think for themselves, but instead is a project of inculcating absolute obedience. A teacher's responsibility is premised on deference to the assumption that one's students come with "fixed" beliefs whose expansion to any degree constitutes an undermining of "parental authority." This helps me to understand the startling fundamentalism reflected in the Nevada Family Alliance's proposal that teachers wear body cameras: it would bring parents into the classroom as virtual overseers, as monitors, as rapporteurs, with permanent transcripts of every word that is spoken.

This would be, to say the least, chilling not only to free speech but to the possibility of young people learning to become independent. It is one thing to put body cams on police officers where life and death decisions are by their very nature the subject of forensic analysis; it is quite a different project to frame student-teacher encounters as the fodder for trial and evidentiary examination in an architecture of litigious surveillance. If teachers cannot be trusted and the classroom becomes a geography of police patrol by nanny cam, the nature of teaching changes and eliminates environments where students might take risks and have the freedom of making mistakes.

Finally, these new laws seem unmoored to any shared sense of limits or definition of *what other than personal distress* would give rise to the ability to fire a teacher whose student became upset. Like pornography, are we supposed to know it when we see it? That amorphousness floats like the heaviest irony over campus culture wars that have sometimes degenerated, like overwrought children's birthday parties, into sophomoric crying jags about who's upsetting whom, who has the right to shut whom up, who's suffered more, who's got the thinnest skin. Those debacles, their usual pettiness, and their often overzealous reactivity, particularly within universities, have long raised concerns among all who work in academia. It's not easy herding cats as they emerge from vastly different home environments—whether they're seven years old, teenagers, or in graduate school. I am not alone in having advocated more Kleenex and more patience in getting through these difficult encounters, the outgrowth of a polity fractured by hothoused hyper-segregation. All those who teach—of all ideologies, right or left, and not just critical race theorists—worry about immature students yelling, crying, and reporting each other as a form of dispute resolution. That much is hardly a new challenge; it comes with the job. Sometimes it can feel like a weirdly dystopic game show, a nation of people (now including politicians) hurling insults at each other with the generous exuberance of Oprah dispensing free cars.

"You're a racist!"

"No, *you're* a racist!"

"And you're a misogynist, too!"

As hard as those moments may be to wade through and resolve, working through them is a far cry from dealing with difficulties by actually outlawing words like *racism*. That is a simple-minded solution stemming from rigidly fundamentalist nonthinking that mistakes a word for the thing it signifies. Words surely have meaning and can summon new worlds; words certainly have the potential force to organize hurtful laws, command actions, or invoke death. That said, the word *stick* is not a stick and the word *stone* is not an actual stone.

It is silly to think that eliminating the word *racism* will eliminate racism's complex history and the resultant network of ruined human encounters. Yet, according to PEN America's Index of School Book Bans, thousands of volumes have been removed from curricula or withheld from libraries since the purge began in 2021.[31]

8
Process of Elimination

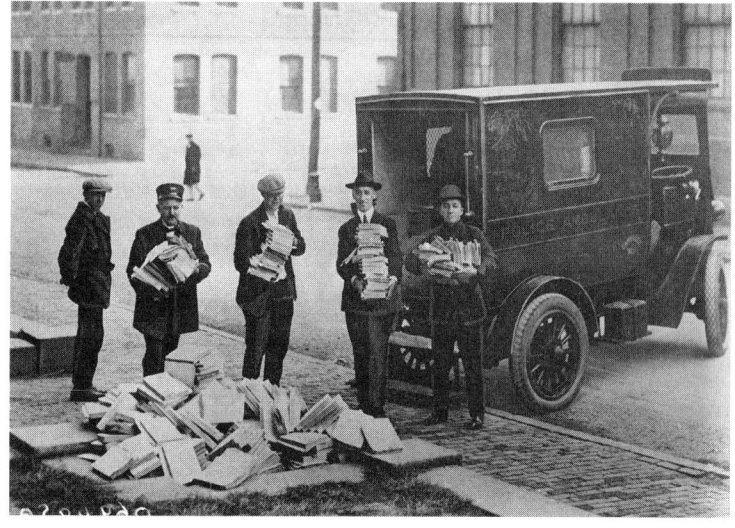

Boston police with piles of communist literature they seized and banned as a precaution against revolution in America

Photo by © Hulton-Deutsch Collection/CORBIS/Corbis via Getty Images

In Florida, the Collier County Public Schools District has affixed a warning label on more than a hundred books, including Toni Morrison's *Beloved*: "This Advisory Notice shall serve to inform you that this book has been identified by some community members as unsuitable for students. This book will also be identified in the Destiny [school library management] system with this same notation. This decision as to whether this book is suitable or unsuitable shall be the decision of the parent(s) who has the right to oversee his/her child's education consistent with state law."[1] This notice tags a book not simply in its physical form on a particular classroom's bookshelf but follows its cyber-manifestation into the eternity of a seemingly unironic Destiny. It suggests that status as "unsuitable for students" may presage a broader and possibly more enduring inaccessibility online.

Even where books are not removed outright from public or school libraries, another alarming form of restriction has sometimes taken hold: the trend toward defunding and/or removing public libraries altogether. In Jamestown, Michigan, citizens voted to defund and close their public library following a push from conservatives to remove a single book from the shelves—*Gender Queer* by Maia Kobabe.[2] In Huntsville, Alabama, the city council voted to privatize the public library by outsourcing management and staffing services to Library Systems and Services, LLC, a for-profit company based in Maryland. This move came after the city librarian was placed on leave, and after a monthslong controversy about the removal of a pride display at the library. The city council cited nothing about the substantive question of book removal; rather, it issued a statement that justified the move entirely in economic and profit-motive terms. The outsourcing would cut costs by 10 percent; it would "increase efficiency" with "a more streamlined process" of "collection development" that would be less "time consuming" and no longer "exhaust staff members' time."[3]

The attacks licensed by laws in Florida, Texas, and other states will affect what all American children in any state will be taught. Textbook publishing is a $4.8 billion business, and Florida is among the biggest customers. In an effort to retain Florida schools as customers, companies have begun to cater to anti–critical race theory laws' restrictions.[4] In March 2023, the *New York Times* looked at what Studies Weekly, whose publications are used in 45,000 schools nationwide, submitted for approval by Florida's new review board since passage of the "Stop WOKE" law in 2022. The *Times* compared three versions of

Studies Weekly's presentation of the history of Rosa Parks. First was the version currently in use in Florida; it reads: "In 1955, Rosa Parks broke the law. In her city, the law said African Americans had to give up their seats on the bus if a white person wanted to sit down. She would not. The police came and took her to jail."

The second version was one initially submitted for the state's new textbook review; it reads: "Rosa Parks showed courage. One day she rode the bus. She was told to move to a different seat because of the color of her skin. She did not. She did what she believed is right."

The third and most recent submission to the review board, however, was revised even more radically, so that neither race nor segregation is mentioned at all: "Rosa Parks showed courage. One day she rode the bus. She was told to move to a different seat. She did not. She did what she believed was right."[5]

Also, according to the *New York Times*, within a year of the Stop WOKE Act's passage, the conservative Florida Citizens Alliance, a private organization that holds great sway with Governor DeSantis, had recommended removal of "28 of the 38 textbooks that its volunteers reviewed, including more than a dozen by McGraw Hill, a major national publisher."[6] It is unclear what metrics are in place other than elimination when it is reported that the Florida Citizens Alliance "complained that a McGraw Hill fifth-grade textbook, for example, mentioned slavery 189 times within a few chapters alone."[7] If the chapters are about slavery, it seems highly reductive to assert that the mere number of times a word is mentioned should determine its educational value—unless the goal is to diminish or excise the topic altogether.

It is worth stressing that book publishing is a business whose profit margin is significantly threatened by states that implement anti-CRT laws. With "rational economic" logic, publishers are incentivized to trim their product in ways that appeal to the broadest audiences possible—i.e., the lowest common denominator. The powerhouse publisher Scholastic Books, for example, recently suggested eliminating the word "racism" from Maggie Tokuda-Hall's story *Love in the Library*, an account of how her grandparents fell in love in an internment camp for Japanese Americans during World War II. The editors wrote her a note stating that it was a "politically sensitive" moment for book marketing and that they did not wish to go "beyond what some teachers are willing to cover with the kids in their elementary classrooms. This could lead to teachers declining to use the book, which would be a shame."[8] As Mokuda-Hall observed, eliminating the historical context of anti-Asian racism reduces it to "just being like a lovely little love story. And that's not what it is. To pretend otherwise would do a disservice not just to [my grandparents], but also to the 120,000 other people who were incarcerated at the time." Scholastic apologized, but Mokuda-Hall worries that despite "a momentary flurry of outrage . . . nothing changes. And other creators are asked to make horrible choices like this going forward in the dark."[9]

I do not know, but I suspect that such profit-motivated "review" of texts—by the publishers as well as the censors—is being conducted by efficient technology that searches for keywords and makes maps of their frequency, with no regard for substance, context, meaning, or message. This problem infects other realms as well, such as hiring: unregulated as this entire field is, some software has been found to scan résumés for membership in ethnic-sounding social clubs, to quietly mark certain zip codes for elimination, or to reject anyone who attended an all-women's college.[10]

Increasingly, we are being quietly normed by the suggestive seductions of quantitative maps—of books, literature, philosophy, ideas. Tools like Voyant and Dreamscape are web scrapers that perform digital text analysis and deliver "word frequency lists, frequency distribution plots, and KWIC displays (KWIC, an acronym for Key Words in Context, is an indexing system that performs database searches tabulating the sequence of words that precede and follow a chosen keyword)."[11] Such tools can generate maps that measure "vocabulary density," number of words, and average number of words per sentence. The most frequently used words in Toni Morrison's novel *Jazz*, for example, are "like," "violet," "said," and "know."[12]

No doubt this is useful as an indexing tool. It's a compelling presentation of information, but substantively neutral with regard to the novel's literary significance. Its quantification is an insignificant part of the project of deriving meaning. Toni Morrison herself observed that: "data" means little without the larger context of "information, knowledge, and wisdom."[13]

Even if specific tools like Dreamscape (packaged as "the hyper-gamified reading program") are not deployed, the increasingly quantitative turn in our ubiquitously data-fied and data-fed thinking means that review of educational materials sometimes tends to skirt substantive assessment in favor of reductive forms of content mapping. Given that cyberspace is predominantly commercial and privatized, the subtler consequences of technology's reorganization of social norms remain largely under-examined. For example, as a teacher, I rue the degree to which academic metrics are being quietly shunted more and more toward the exclusively quantitative. Zoom and Canvas, and the universities purchasing their services, usually assert ownership rights to any teaching material—including lectures recorded on those sites—thus forcing teachers to provide salable content for the platform corporations.

In another example, Perusall is an e-reader platform that allows students to annotate assigned reading, highlight sections, write notes, and discuss the material with one another. It grades each student based not merely on the substantive pertinence of their commentary, but on the *number* of annotations, and on *time* spent on active reading. For each reading, students receive a grade determined by Perusall's algorithm. In other words, one's individual reading habits must be made transparent to the machine: one is effectively discredited for time spent reading the book in a nontrackable forum, e.g., the print version. One is even penalized if one is a fast reader. Indeed, one is potentially rewarded for being a slowly lingering reader.

"Information" or extracted data, seems to possess a much higher value than knowledge or wisdom. That reductiveness makes me think of an old cartoon by Roz Chast from the *New Yorker*. Captioned "The Tree of Information," it shows the snake leaning down from a branch proffering an apple to Eve. "The apple is a tree fruit," he says. "Its Latin name is Malus domestica. China and the U.S. produce most of the world's apples. It can be eaten raw or cooked, and contains about 75 calories."

Teachers, too—or anyone who uses computers for work—are increasingly valued by the data that can be made legible to the quantifications of artificial intelligence. Microsoft Viva sends me regular reports complaining about my productivity: it tells me I have not been sufficiently detailed in terms of how I allocate "time for myself." It assures me I will be more efficient if I enter all my daily, hourly, minute-by-minute appointments, meetings, and obligations onto their server. Something called MyAnalytics feeds me a weekly list of people with whom I've had online encounters. It ranks them by frequency of contact. It reports whether I've sent any email during online meetings; it reports how many times I've spoken during a particular meeting, and how often I've participated in chat-room conversations during those meetings. It tells me that I must schedule more of my life in ways legible to MyAnalytic—because "it"—that passive invisible "it"—makes negative value judgments about time it frowns upon as "unallocated." MyAnalytic nudges me to "increase personal productivity" by revealing, feeding more of my daily activities into the maw of its hungry, hungry database. Thinking, listening, or quiet unrecorded reflection seems to be dismissed as "inutility," quietly ushered out of the project of constructive thought. This Taylorist transformation of social relation—whether in grading practices or creative production—is largely unquestioned even as it imposes quietly disruptive and sternly anti-democratic norms.

When I was in high school, decades before the internet, we had something that we called Facebook. It was a big notebook, made of paper, with two cardboard covers. I went to school with a very skilled cadre of Mean Girls, so every year in the beginning of the year, the social hierarchy would be set by *that book*, that Facebook version sub-one, pre–Mac Pro, with a memory capacity of fifty loose-leaf pages. It would be secretively handed from person to person, up and down the aisles during Latin class. Each student's name was written at the top of a page, and underneath people would enter anonymous opinions about that person. The opinions were creative and detailed and because they were anonymous, they were cruel. Exceptionally cruel. And if, as so often happened to me, if the book was handed over your head—if it bypassed you, if your access was denied—then you knew that what was said about you was too terrible even to share. You knew that you had been terminally unfriended.

Flash forward to the present. I don't know whether Mark Zuckerberg got the name Facebook from that primitive but fairly ubiquitous teenage rating game, but I'm old enough to remember when that's all it meant. There are rumors that Zuckerberg's first product, created when he was in college, was called FaceMash, an app for ranking women as "hot-or-not."[14] To me, today's multibillion-dollar version of Facebook remains a sophomoric instrument of revenge, a device amplifying the high school hardcopy Facebook, seamlessly manipulating the teenage desire to be liked, the nerd's fear of missing out, the threat of being excluded from the room of many likes. The architecture of this technology is through one lens a really simple business model, but it's also a psychic trap on steroids. It appeals to human longing to belong, but it cultivates loneliness; we connect in isolation. Algorithmic networks are powerful but oxymoronic: plural but solitary, intimate but remote. We exist, especially now, enclosed in numbers, our bodies conveyed as tile renderings, trapped as though in a cult by rule of others' opinions.

Perhaps the sudden crises presented by the recent years of political polarization have finally foregrounded the dangers lurking in the ultra-libertarian shrug of "I have nothing to hide"—that mantra one heard in the early days of internet surveillance. "It's so convenient," remains the insistent justification for algorithmic assortments that serve us up suggestions for the perfect book, the perfect recipe, the perfect game. It is all but impossible to function in a contemporary economy without such "efficient" surveillance, without an assortment of phones, watches, and other tracking devices attached to our bodies like demonic little leeches disguised as smiling, servile, nearly invisible helpmeets. But as our machines fatten themselves on gluttonous feasts of our data, it is increasingly clear that living in a technological panopticon makes us vulnerable to corporate manipulations that equate due process with business inefficiency and dismiss algorithmic transparency as an infringement of trade secrets.

Just so, revenge porn, algorithmic bias, and identity theft have become all-too-common experiences. Data culled from commercial databases have enabled new forms of granular tracking in a time when heated passions fuel inquisitions that can amount to harassment and endangerment—of teachers, journalists, census takers, bookstores, voters, poll watchers, librarians, accountants with the Internal Revenue Service, public health workers, doctors, nurses, judges, ex-spouses, and now even FBI agents—anyone deemed guilty of an ever expanding list of activities targeted as the errancy of the moment.

Made particularly obvious in the wake of the Supreme Court's overturning *Roe v. Wade*, digital tracking poses invasive and dehumanizing peril for millions of Americans. Heretofore, only a few Americans seemed to grasp that supposedly "private" information collected by apps that track menstrual cycles might be sold to—as well as hacked and scraped by—private vigilantes determined to follow the activities of potentially pregnant women. Moreover, new statutes criminalizing abortion have empowered police departments to use individual citizens' social media data to file charges against women who may have ordered medications like abortion pills mailed to them across state lines. In one recent case, police in Nebraska issued a warrant for the Facebook communications between a mother and her teenage daughter, revealing that the daughter had taken a mail-ordered abortifacient and, as a result, miscarried at twenty-two weeks.[15] Prosecutors charged the mother with "performing an abortion without a medical license," and attempting to abort a fetus more than twenty weeks old. Her seventeen-year-old daughter, charged as an adult, was accused of mishandling human remains and failing to report a death.

The architecture of this surveillance technology has reconfigured what we are used to thinking of as governance: our constitutional right to privacy is jurisprudentially rooted in a tradition of autonomy and interiority that was historically styled as a region of dignity, bounded against intrusion by the state. But state structures of surveillance have been vastly overtaken by the internet's evolution as a predominantly commercial space, with infinite profit motive for unfettered intrusion; there is ungoverned bounty for data grabbing. The supposed notice and consent proffered by the "I agree" buttons we press to access any given platform is woefully ineffective as a mechanism imparting anything like choice. Yet that empty assurance of "choice" is the vocabulary used to justify information-gathering practices about everything from our voting preferences to bathroom habits to musical tastes to blood pressure and sleep patterns. Despite vague promises that such data is "anonymized," it can be bought, sold, scraped, reassembled, reidentified, and used to home in on particular individuals with laser-like predictive precision about specific behaviors. Moreover, because giant social media platforms are not officially state actors, we can't easily summon the same causes of action against them, for censorship or denial of public accommodation. As private, corporate, profit-seeking businesses, they are responsible only to their shareholders. Our human vulnerabilities are of relevance to these companies only as consumers in a market economy, not as citizens in a diverse social network. And if we decline their terms of service, we are caught in a double bind, a "voluntary choice" that involuntarily excludes us from basic life necessities: credit cards, cell phones, banking transactions, workplace duties, insurance, credit rating, schooling, shopping, health services, housing.

This collective re-norming to accommodate the voyeuristic, 24/7, know-it-all appetites of Big Data is oppressive. In 2022, when Sanna Marin, who was the Finnish prime minister at the time, was filmed dancing at a party with friends, a great deal of ink was spilled evaluating her behavior for conduct unbecoming a prime minister; for exuberance indicative of having been possibly excited by illicit drug use; and for failing to "restrain herself in company where she cannot trust everyone in the room."[16] That framing puts the onus on her, however—and on each of us as individuals to closely monitor ourselves even in closed rooms. It structures us perpetually to distrust weddings, birthday parties—anywhere there are others who have cell phones. It locates the "fault" of the video's circulation as a matter of individual intentionality and restricts our imagination to carelessness and "leaks." One cybersecurity expert "raised the possibility Russia had hacked the phone or social accounts of someone who is part of the close circle of the Finnish premier."[17]

It should be remembered that Marin was in a supposedly private space at a supposedly private party. Technology being what it is, it didn't have to be an overtly intentional exposure. Yes, it could have been an undercover Russian spy, or a celebrity stalker paid off to share dirt. But it is just as possible that a real friend posted it—for supposedly "personal use"—on Facebook, or WhatsApp or TikTok. It is too easy to forget that nothing posted on those platforms is ever really personal—even in the European Union, which has somewhat stronger protections than the United States. This kind of inadvertent surveillance is always a problem when posting content for supposedly "personal" use. It can be extracted and exploited for both legal and illegal ends: to threaten political careers, to defame and embarrass, or, as we see in red states, to threaten women who are thinking about—or who are thought to be thinking about—abortion, contraception, or other "disobedience" in our brave new world.

One does not have to be a celebrity or prime minister to worry about such intrusive exposure. Recently, a friend related that she'd stopped going to her favorite gym class because someone repeatedly pulled out a cell phone and filmed the class without seeking permission. The gym had a clear statement in its membership rules: "Photography and videography strictly prohibited." But when she objected, she found no recourse: not just the people wielding the cameras, but the teacher and other members of the class dismissed her with three primary assertions: 1. "It's just for personal use." 2. She was of a "different generation," so her objections could be ignored, even laughed at. 3. If she wanted "privacy," she should find a class online. There is an entanglement of contradictory expectations in those responses to her concerns: first, that anything recorded on a cell phone can or will be constrained as exclusively "personal." Second, that capturing her image for someone else's "personal" use without consent is fine, dandy, no harm done, and not even her "business." Third, that she shouldn't take the possibility of her image being published so seriously—that "you're not that important."

This experience raises other concerns in the context of the Federal Trade Commission's failure to regulate commercial surveillance. Does the refusal to govern cell phone camera usage turn gyms and a range of other venues into unwalled public spaces despite stated membership rules or conventions of decorum? Or, if you don't want other people filming you, must the default resolution be such a narrowly libertarian one—to wit, an individual burden to remove oneself from such risky social contexts and just retreat to the (no less risky) burrow of "online" connectivity? Must we really allow the casual commerce of selfies (using muted others as vanity backdrops) to override even explicit contractual terms? What diminishment does this impose on the notion of public accommodation, supposedly inherent in the notion of shared space? Does my friend's unhappiness have any social purchase as deserving the respect necessary in being among others, as a claim for mutual restraint, deference, or negotiation due in any gathering anywhere? And what might any of us want as a gentle behavioral norm in ambiguously intimate spaces like a gym class? What trust might be violated by surveillance technologies that broadcast that space to unseen others beyond those walls?

My friend described the ineffability of her melancholy at some length:

> I know I'm not a celebrity. I'm not really important enough for anyone to care. But it's exactly because I'm so irrelevant to those young people living in their video'd fantasy worlds that I felt so vulnerable and so incidental. In cardio class, I give myself permission to get hot, sweaty, happy, goofy. I know I'm not fit for general inspection, bouncing around, shaking my booty, trying to keep my heartrate at peak level. I go to the gym to try to feel better about myself the next day, not to be captured in the moment with my mascara dripping down my face like Rudy Guiliani's hair dye. Images like that follow you. Being filmed for someone else's "personal use" makes me feel even more out of control of my life than I already do. Maybe I'm just a control freak. Maybe this just brings back the humiliation of high school gym classes. But I honestly think I'm like a lot of people, who are older, out-of-shape, or somewhat disabled. I'm also a woman

whose public-facing day job requires wearing sensible suits and maintaining a professional demeanor. My work presentation is in complete contrast to when I let loose to the thumping beat of Bruno Mars. I don't think I'm alone in feeling betrayed in that setting, betrayed by random photographic exposure. I think of gym membership as a safe space for getting in shape, not as a theatrical backdrop for others' vanity pics. That's the whole reason for the *rule* against taking pictures.

My friend's experience also underscores the significant generational shift that has occurred just within the last several years. As recently as ten or fifteen years ago, most people would not have dreamed of taking pictures in a gym without permission. There was, I think, a stronger set of social conventions about averting one's eyes from others' daily rituals, embarrassments, ablutions, and purifications. This generational divergence around manners is not only a matter of chronological age, though. Even more significantly, it's evidence of a shift in ideological constructs, the growth of a crassly libertarian, tech-inflected disposition that turns even public space into visual fields that may be divvied up, manipulated, and exploited for viral titillation and the self-aggrandizement of accumulated "likes"—even if at the thoughtless expense of others who may be present within that space. Admittedly, this is a phenomenon that implicates manners more than what law may be able to resolve; it is the unintended consequence of technology that not only connects the world, but hands a bully pulpit to outright bullies. Nevertheless, the pervasive lack of self-regulation overtakes public space and endangers the very notion of civility.

This tabloidization of everything was on display in 2016, when, late one night in New York City, a man began taking a video of the near-empty subway car in which he was riding. He was filming a large rat scuttling along the length of the car. When the rat proceeded to climb onto a sleeping fellow passenger, the man continued to film. "So I see the rat crawl onto the guy, and zoomed in," was his description of the sequence of events. He zoomed in to capture the rat scampering all the way up to the sleeping man's shoulder. Our brave videographer quickly hid his cellphone when, after a nuzzle to the ear, the man woke up screaming. But then, just as quickly, the cameraman posted the video on Instagram, summing up his feelings to the global press as follows: "It's just insane and disgusting overall to see that."[18] "SEE IT," wrote the *New York Daily News*.[19] "Watch It," wrote NBC.[20]

To me, the most interesting part of this story was the oddly clandestine tension felt by the man who filmed it but who then felt no hesitation about publicizing it. He said he panicked when the man woke up; he hid the camera because he didn't want to be seen watching and seeing. One must wonder why? Was it out of regard for the sleeping man's now breached privacy? Was he hiding the camera as a way of acknowledging some felt zone of privacy that attends someone sleeping in public? Was it guilt? I can't imagine passively watching a rat climb on someone without trying to do something, like yell loudly, or some other effort either to wake the sleeper or to frighten off the rat. It is intriguing: What sense of propriety was at stake in that moment of unwillingness to be seen "taking" pictures? Was it the fear of actual human encounter with the object of his memorializing? Was it a sudden realization that his titillation at the "insane and disgusting" was also someone else's experience of abject terror and humiliation?

Selfies are only the most conspicuous expression of a laissez-faire culture that is, just as the name implies, all about the self rather than others. It ennobles the gaze of the monetized "influencer" for whom the mirrored self is alpha and omega. I also think it reflects a juridical transformation. The privatized commercial value of data now tends to govern outcome much more than collective or public interests, including law. Legal rules can too often be overridden in the free-for-all that is the ungoverned power usurped by the camera, the platform, by Google or ATT or Facebook. The burden is on singular individuals to figure out the labyrinthine rules in the terms of agreement; it's up to the lonely you to scour those terms every day, every moment. Most standardized contracts clearly state they can change the terms of agreement and all those privacy expectations without your "further" consent or notice. In other words, when one takes a picture and sends it to someone on Facebook or WhatsApp or Instagram or TikTok, one's "intention" that it be only for "personal use" is a hollow expectation, for we have delivered our secrets to a predatory behemoth.

However it was that Prime Minister Marin's happy dance became viral, it shouldn't be a surprise. We are all at risk of being decontextualized through revelation of unguarded moments. Our worth in the office is not limited to what we do *in* the office. Social media has become an unforgiving monitor of our slightest indiscretions, even in the bedroom. While we, the public, may hold each other to norms of the sober, industrious, and dignified in the workplace, tracking each other behind closed doors and during off-hours has become a monetized game of gotcha, an eternal reality show that rewrites the notion of an open society into a tyranny of voyeurs and outright pornographers.

And still, we seem largely oblivious: we wander through the metaverse like Little Red Riding Hood. We are innocent; our path through the forest *feels* like a secret. We don't worry—we don't imagine the existence of the wolves who track our happy trajectory. We hum as we proceed, distracted by milkweed blossoms, the aroma of warm cookies, and the promise of a good sale at Walmart. But where does the knowledge of our secret meandering go? Who follows our familiar paths, our inner whimsy? How thin is the scrim that separates any of us—in any context—from the armchair censure of millions of strangers, the context collapse that occurs when precious bits of ourselves are viewed by multiple audiences situated at multiple distances, in multiple cultural contexts? Who are we when the intimacy of immediate or intimate context is unconsidered, lost, unknown—or sold down a river of infobits? For the most part, we exist in these cyber worlds ignorant as lambs, helpless as babes, unarmed as fish in a barrel, innocent as kittens tossed down the well. We are collateral in the market for data, even when tracked, trolled, misread, targeted, stripped, mocked, harassed, humiliated, bankrupted, our naked images photoshopped in some subreddit: all are mere transaction costs to the hungry leviathan that devours our every move and extracts monetary value from it that we will never know.

In the Netflix film *The Social Dilemma*, Cathy O'Neill, author of *Weapons of Math Destruction*, is quoted as saying "algorithms are opinions embedded in code . . . then optimized to some definition of success." And so we live in a world where the equivalent of trillions of cyber-mean girls have been let loose, hooked up with advertisers and monopolized commercial interests and extreme ideologues and professional manipulators, not to mention pornographers and warmongers.

The granularity of present data extraction is not only about monetization of personal privacy; it also creates the sort of surveillance system that, as a child of the Cold War, I was taught to fear and associate with the KGB. We read about Stalin and the temperamental Mr. Khrushchev; we read of the experiences of exiled novelists and dancers and athletes who fled to the West from behind the Iron Curtain. The USSR, we were told, was oppressive because of its system of secret police, inhuman gulags, and lack of due process. It is therefore quite astonishing to wake up and find the Bill of Rights effectively upended by the uses of data to conform our civic lives based on calculations of a war on terror whose assessments seem to proceed from broad assumptions that, as Orwell put it, "whatever goes on two legs is an enemy." Not only are citizens not "secure in their papers," as the Fourth Amendment puts it; neither are they secure in their computers, cell phones, global positioning chips, medical histories, credit cards, nannycams, heartbeat tracking devices, or DNA trails. In a land where everyone's a suspect, there's probable cause to search everyone.

Such high-tech voyeurism has any number of unsettling consequences, not least of which is that Calvinist notions like the doctrine of total depravity seem to have displaced the legal presumption of innocence. Increasingly, one sees ubiquitous CCTV, indefinite detention, and strip searches of schoolchildren "justified" as checks upon humanity's presumptively inherent transgressivity.

Creative accommodation to totalistic oversight is even written into our very sense of time. As philosopher Brian Massumi stated in his critique of the circular logic of the invasion of Iraq: "The invasion was right because in the past there was a future threat." Just so, policies based on ethics of diplomacy, equity, healing, and peace among the nations of the Earth are increasingly brushed aside, treated as seductive plots to lure the naive into settling for heathenish relativism and letting down one's guard. As Massumi continues, "Self-renewing menace potential is the future reality of threat. . . . The future of threat is forever." The sense of divine inevitability that informs this civic vision allows us to wash our hands of a whole raft of otherwise obvious political and religious injunctions: feed the poor, heal the sick, educate the illiterate, house the homeless, rehabilitate the wounded, give shelter to asylum seekers. George Orwell feared communism, fascism, totalitarianism, and all their attendant linguistic conceits. What he did not foresee, perhaps, was a global distribution of private eyes, a fragmented and unaccountable police power wrapped in the sheep's clothing of laissez-faire.

9
Roots

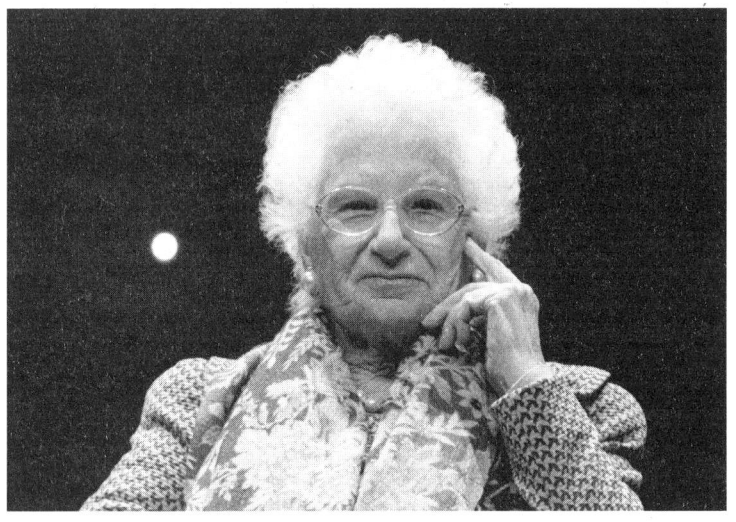

Giorgio Perottino/Getty Images

Liliana Segre, born in 1930, is an Italian life senator and survivor of the Holocaust. She heads a parliamentary commission to combat racism, antisemitism, and incitement to hatred. It is sadly ironic that Segre, who was the only member of her family to escape Auschwitz, has lived long enough to become the oldest person in Europe to have a police escort. Since 2019, she has received increasing numbers of death threats for her anti-racism work, and more recently, for her work supporting COVID vaccines. "Living under a police escort at the age of 92 is unbelievable," she says. "I have been subjected to racist attacks, unbelievable things. It's never face-to-face; everything is consumed and amplified online—a closed place where keyboard haters unleash the worst of human instincts with authentic brutality, with their faces covered and identities disguised as pet names."[1]

It is surely true that rapidly expanding technological abilities to connect and "correct" our minds and bodies have brought vast efficiencies and benefits. That power is one of unprecedented social transformation and reorganization. At the same time, it is a power that has been coopted by only a few individuals, largely invisible and hugely unaccountable. Willingly or inadvertently, consumers and regulatory agencies have ceded control to monopolies and private ownership. Massive global entities like Twitter, Facebook, and Google are governed by a handful of individuals with little transparency and no instincts for democracy, fairness, or mercy. With the amplified logics of the parable with which I began this book, to wit, Shannon Whisnant's commodification of John Wood's embalmed leg, a small boy band of billionaire technocrats has commandeered an astonishing power of surveillance over every place we go, every friend we make, every breath we take. With that universal corporate tech comes the power to play with our emotions, nudge our decision making, monitor our resentments, inflame our desires, invade our bedrooms, steer our job options, measure our heartbeats, publicize our secrets, dictate our medical treatment, silence our complaints, and restrict our ability to find address and redress. Such techno-totalitarianism is like having all of life reduced to a page in my high school version of Facebook. We face the existential conundrum of being locked in solitary confinement while simultaneously overexposed to millions of other people's opinions, nibbling away at our thoughts and our bodies like schools of piranhas.

This model has been allowed to enter our brains, take over our thoughts, and addict us to riding the wave of constant, consuming, instantaneous information. We are so consumed that we are starved in every other realm of existence; we don't eat, we don't sleep, we don't touch, we don't breathe, we don't move. This merging with a quantitative composite of ourselves has taken over the space within us where our most healing sensations of humanity used to reside. It has entered and occupied the generative domain of trance, ritual, and daydream, subverting the exclusivities of both private ownership and public domain. Everything comes to us from an outside that feels internal to ourselves, that defines us, leads us, in this so-called "attention-distraction extraction model."[2] One great cost would seem to be that our political will—our capacity for civic participation—has been vitiated accordingly, rendered harder to focus, distracted and abstracted, as well as extracted. In her book *Thinking in an Emergency*, Elaine Scarry writes that the "abridging of rights and laws more often lacks any sensory manifestation."[3]

I thought about this recently when a parade passed in the street beneath the window of my office. Several hundred people marched by bearing banners and bullhorns. They had only two chants: "Shame! Shame! Shame!" and "We say *no*!" But what was interesting was that the object of the protest was unstated as far as I could tell. It could have been about so many things—masks, no masks, vaccinations, no vaccinations, abortion rights, abortion wrongs, critical race theory, no critical race theory, the war in Ukraine, the war in Congo, inflation, energy prices, voting or the lack thereof. I even wondered if the absence of stated cause was in artful counterpoint to recent losses of freedom of expression exemplified by the banning of thousands of books in schools and libraries across the country.

As the list of possibilities scrolled through my mind, however, I began to suppose that the protest may not have needed an "about." The apparent aimlessness of that march could well have been the point. Perhaps the moral panic of it was the point. The shame-shame-shaming was the point. Oppositional defiance was perhaps the order of the day and this was loud theater about being silenced. The fill-in-the-blank nature of their noisy shouting made me think of those in Russia who have protested harsh censorship laws by holding up posters that are entirely blank—and have then been jailed for even that much-too-powerfully expressive wordlessness.

If libertarianism is built into the machine as a driver of the profit motive upon which tech markets feed, perhaps emotions like fear and distrust may be as well. Algorithms learn from and replicate the emotional state of their architects, the human programmers, for artificial intelligence is only as interesting as the data upon which it is trained. Even highly sophisticated and improvisational large-language modeling systems—including chatbots like ChatGPT—are norming machines, assortative devices that determine identity mostly via binarisms rooted in one thing being like or not like another. This is how some systems have famously mistaken an image of a peach for naked human buttocks. Or how a self-driving car can mistake the setting sun for a stoplight.

There is a literalism to artificial intelligence that is surely correctable, but in subtler social classifications and typologizing, it may evade correction merely because the machine's mistakes reflect the norms of its human programmer parents. Moreover, once such programs become sold as commodities or put into so-called black boxes, they are often very hard to open back up for recalibration. The problems of black-box decision making are well documented in Virginia Eubanks's excellent book *Automated Inequality*.[4] When complex human assessments of bail, parole, or child custody are made based on the basis of probabilistic, quantitative weighting, grave injustices may occur in the name of statistical consistency of outcome. A machine cannot take into account any individual circumstances that it has not been trained to see during its manufacture. Moreover, black-box calculations do not ordinarily grant a right of review or appeal. Unlike the analysis of a judge or a social worker, the interstices of the algorithmic reasoning process are frequently impossible to know.

The degree to which algorithmic mistakes replicate the prejudices of actuarial practice generally was revealed when researchers in California found that calculations for prisoners' parole worthiness were in part based on zip code.[5] In other words, "neighborhood" was weighted more heavily than the behavior, accomplishments, or rehabilitation of a particular individual. The algorithm was incorporating a notion of neighborhood as a cipher for class, race, and/or occurrence of criminality and then punishing individuals for programmers' biases about certain geographies, thus creating zones of inevitable civil death.

In short, the problem is not that processors can't replicate human intelligence, but that they *can* all too accurately replicate human prejudice, substituting plurals for singulars and singulars for plurals. It is the risk of all stereotyping: the mistaking of probabilities for foregone conclusions.

Algorithmic decision making merely replicates and magnifies a basic problem of language, not all that different from how to assign value to John Wood's leg: holy relic or Halloween horror? The difficulty is, again, a discursive problem of naming practices, situational ethics, indexical relation, and deictic pattern recognition.

Algorithms name as well as assort, and in that process they may inscribe forms of categoric fundamentalism—which is how I became known as Hot Cheeto Girl among a certain circle of acquaintances. There I was at a yoga retreat, innocently eating my lunch, consisting of grilled octopus, edamame, sesame noodles . . . and a bag of Flamin' Hot Cheetos. A young friend tilted her head in curiosity and told me that I was such an inscrutable oddball. I thought she was referring to the octopus, which might mark me as rather Whole Foods-y. But she was fixated upon those Cheetos. I was, in her youthful lexicon of memes, an unusually elderly example of a Hot Cheeto Girl. I was a curiosity to her because I didn't quite fit the mold, couldn't easily be squeezed into the box. I had to look it up later, for it's actually a thing: according to the online Urban Dictionary, a Hot Cheeto "girl" (I am not even a Hot Cheeto "woman"!) is the loud one "in the back of the classroom who is always snacking on hot cheetos or takis. Usually a woman of color (mainly Hispanic or Black), Hot Cheeto girls wear thrasher shirts, checkered vans and ripped jeans. They can be seen with their hair in a large bun and their edges done. They usually have long acrylic nails . . . and are always ready to fight a bitch."[6]

On the one hand, the description was infantile and absurdly risible. On the other, I realize that I purchased those Hot Cheetos with my credit card, so that somewhere in my social media profile there is most likely a little algorithm that has me pegged.

It is an odd feeling to be dispossessed of one's body. I float above the trillion data points that mark the thing I call myself, simultaneously digital and disconnected, the head empty with light, the skin too tight, the heart too dark, too full. I want to appear, I want the body electric. It shimmers past me, gossamer, translucent, ineffable, untouchable. It is impossible to read myself, a face that has been booked. Voice, vocals, verbiage, and visuals all play against one another, rather than together. The elements refuse to fuse, they float away, thin air, destabilizing bits.

I suppose I need translation. There are parts of me that signify outside my understanding—my hands, my voice, my mismatched eyes, my dead white hair.

I think about my own muddled attempts at assigning category. Some years ago, I was trying to count the number of African American students in my son's class. "Let me see . . . ," I said. "There's you and A and B and C . . .

C's not Black, he said.

I was surprised. I knew C, her parents, and her grandparents. By most societal measures, they would be thought of as Black. So I asked: "Why do you say that?"

She hangs out with the white kids.

"And you don't? What about your three best friends, X, Y, and Z?"

They're Black.

"All three of them are quite blond! What makes them Black?"
They hang out with me.
"So why aren't you white for hanging out with them, like C?"
Because white kids go to Starbucks and order light Frappuccinos.
"I go to Starbucks!"
And you're white. That's why I don't hang out with you.
"But you go to Starbucks!"
Only twice, and then I ordered a dark chocolate mocha latte.

My son was joshing; he's always playing me. But even as this conversation made me laugh, it also made me think. I was organizing his classmates by some combination of phenotype, family history, and culture. My interest in keeping such a tally was motivated by a wish that my son not be tokenized. Being "the only one" sparks my own anxieties about having grown up as the lone "colored" kid throughout elementary school. In high school, there were a few more dark dots in the mix, which was better because those in the majority couldn't generalize about you quite so easily. And if they did generalize, at least you had someone to roll your eyes with at the absurdity of being lumped together. We fought for inclusiveness in a world that too often hoards life's rewards by racial attribution.

In contrast, my son's social construction of race reminded me of how protean this all is. If it's amusing to think of Starbucks as racial arbiter, it would have been less funny if the racial arbiter had been a brand of sneakers, or a particular accent, or whether one is well educated or not—in other words, if the reference had been to either fixed or negative assumptions about phenotype or class.

There's a lovely quote from Saidiya Hartman's remarkable book *Lose Your Mother*.[7] As she wends her way through Ghana on a Ford Foundation grant, she notes, "I was the stranger in the village, a wandering seed bereft of the possibility of taking root. Behind my back people whispered, *dua ho mmire*: a mushroom that grows on the tree has no deep soil. Everyone avoided the word "slave," but we all knew who was who. As a "slave baby," I represented what most chose to avoid: the catastrophe that was our past. . . . And what was forbidden to discuss: the matter of someone's origins." As I read Hartman's words, I wondered how familiar that sentiment felt to me, or to so many African Americans, whether or not they've ever left our shores or traveled the world; we are always so relentlessly in search of "home." I wondered how familiar that sense of being "out of place" on the planet must feel to human categories in a time of such diaspora. Not long ago, I met a Swedish woman who is phenotypically "Asian." When she was a student in California, she went to the hospital for stomach pains and was almost committed as insane before she ever got to see a doctor. The administrative gatekeepers simply could not reconcile her appearance and her assertion of Swedish citizenship.

I think a lot about the medical consequences of such typecasting as the world rushes to automate its biases. I think of a friend with whom I was in first grade. She used to call me her Best Black Friend. I cured her of that, years later, but still, after a lifetime of valiant trying on both our parts, she retains the power to startle. There we were, having a perfectly amiable chat about actor James Earl Jones's lusciously resonant baritone when she said, "It must be because of the way Black people's larynxes are shaped. You can hear the difference in how their vocal cords affect sound." I was so taken aback by her sudden slippage into an imaginary plural that I could not speak. She saw that I was struggling. "It's probably why you have such a beautiful voice," she added gently, as though application of the aggregate singular might help.

I have been thinking a lot about my friend over the course of these last tumultuous, pandemic-riled years. We are obviously all derailed by the catastrophe of COVID-19, no matter what our relative privilege or status. As another friend described it, it's like going through a car wash without a car; we are being slapped by physical, political, institutional, and financial crises faster than our poor, autonomous organisms can handle. *Wap, wap, wap, wap, those flapping smacking wet rags of doom and death and oh god, here comes the hot wax.* . . .

Some groups are indisputably harder hit than others, however, and what might have slid by as small prejudices in less freighted times now becomes more menacing, even deadly. Racial assumptions shape, predict, and confine all our bodies. The consequences range from silly social outcomes—someone doesn't think I sound "Black enough"— to overt physical peril imposed by distorted fears of biologized Black difference, particularly when such fears are held by police, doctors, teachers, and politicians. COVID-19 has brought home the significance of even casually malign social regard; it has too-well highlighted the housing, health, and economic fissures that divide us. Widespread contagion seems to have isolated us and driven us farther apart from one another, rather than rallying us together in the name of public health. A significant quantum of public health policy was thrown to the winds in favor of saving one's own skin and the titanic efficiencies of a sinking ship. We doomscroll the probabilities of our own survival.

In my own indulgence of doomscrolling, I came across an online article whose title was something like "Do Black Women Matter?" And since I happen to be *a Black Woman*, I wanted to know the answer to that question. I thought I had marked the article in my browser, but I lost it somehow. In my search for it, I turned to Google. I still didn't find it, but instead a boatload of articles popped up that led me to conclude that if Black women do matter, it's not in the way I might have hoped. The Google search referred me to questions addressing why it is that Black women's breasts produce chocolate-colored milk, and why it is that Black women's hair feels like steel when you touch it, and why Black women don't seem to like it when strangers touch their hair without asking, and why it is that Black women have high blood pressure, and how it is that Black women don't get breast cancer or skin cancer, and why Black women have more testosterone than white women, and maybe all that extra testosterone is how come Black women are just so strong, and by the way, why *don't* Black women like you touching their hair? . . . I just don't understand. . . .

There's enough of such nonsense online to really drive home how enduring the ugly normative consequences of slavery remain as profoundly unscientific beliefs in biological difference. Against that depressing backdrop, it's no wonder that there is debate about why Black people are (in fact) dying of COVID in disproportionate numbers, and why Black women are (in fact) dying at greater rates than white women even when they are "just so strong"; and "maybe it's all just genetic" because, you know, their bodies are so Inherently Different . . . In fact: there's a lot of incoherence in the intersection between what we don't know about the virus and what we are just plain ignorant about as social factors.[8]

Then, of course, there's the history. Consider just one well-worn example of how race and science intertwine in what we Americans teach each other: the 1925 case of *State of Tennessee v. John Thomas Scopes*. Scopes was a high school teacher prosecuted for violating the state's Butler Act of 1925, which banned public school teachers from teaching "any theory that denies the Story of Divine Creation of man as taught in the Bible and to teach instead that man has descended from a lower order of animals."[9] The law's rationale was premised on fundamentalist dogma that Biblical literalism transcended all human knowledge. That trial, best known as the Scopes Monkey Trial, is mostly remembered as a battle between science and pseudoscience, but it was also a battle between theological and secular justifications for notions of racial superiority. William Jennings Bryan, arguing for the creationist state law, resisted evolutionary theories that purported to teach children that mankind was descended "not even from American monkeys, but old world monkeys."[10]

While Clarence Darrow is remembered arguing on the more "liberal" side against the Butler Act, the deeper truth is that the secular beliefs of the time were not a lot better than the religious doctrine. The particular theory of evolution Scopes was accused of teaching came from *Civic Biology*, a textbook written by George William Hunter. Hunter wrongly believed, as many do to this day, that there were five distinct human races, representing an ascending order of evolution and civilization: Ethiopian, Malay, American Indian, Mongolian, and Caucasian. He was an enthusiastic defender of segregating each of the five, consistent with the tenets of the then-burgeoning American Eugenics Society and the theories of the infamous eugenicist Charles Davenport. Here's an excerpt from Hunter's textbook prescribing anti-miscegenation as a bulwark against racial "degeneracy":

> Improvement of Man.—If the stock of domesticated animals can be improved, it is not unfair to ask if the health and vigor of the future generations of men and women on the earth might not be improved by applying to them the laws of selection.
>
> The Remedy.—If such people were lower animals, we would probably kill them off to prevent them from spreading. Humanity will not allow this, but we do have the remedy of separating the sexes in asylums or other places and in various ways preventing intermarriage and the possibilities of perpetuating such a low and degenerate race.

The textbook also warned of "Parasitism and its Cost to Society," denouncing "degenerates" and the "feeble-minded," deemed to be "spreading disease, immorality, and crime to all parts of this country. The cost to society of such families is very severe. Largely for them the poorhouse and the asylum exist."

Darrow lost the case, and today we are still fighting about whether creationism may be taught in public schools.

An important aside: Not coincidentally, Williams Jennings Bryan was a good friend of Bob Jones, the evangelist who founded the eponymous Bob Jones University in 1927, in part because of Bryan's urging. Until 1971, Bob Jones University barred admission to African Americans, and offered only limited admission to other minorities. Then, in 1971, under pressure from the Civil Rights Movement, it began to admit only married African Americans. In 1975, after further pressure, it allowed entrance of unmarried African Americans but still forbade interracial dating, and denied entry to "applicants engaged in an interracial marriage or known to advocate interracial marriage or dating." In 1983, the U.S. Supreme Court revoked the university's tax-exempt status based on its racially discriminatory policies. Despite this, the university resisted, based on assertions that God commanded separation of the races. And so it paid several million in back taxes and continued its exclusionary practices based on its freedom of expression under the First Amendment. It continued that policy until 2000, when George W. Bush kicked off his presidential campaign at Bob Jones University. The media uproar prompted its president, Bob Jones III, to nullify the ban on interracial dating, if not on religious grounds, then so as not to haunt Bush's campaign.

Since *Brown v. Board of Education* and then the Civil Rights Act of 1964, American jurisprudence has drawn a distinction between public and private realms in pursuit of policies ensuring nondiscriminatory public access to basic services. Public funds may be withdrawn from schools, businesses, and institutions that engage in forms of invidious discrimination that compromise or threaten the notion of public accommodation. Since the revocation of Bob Jones University's tax-exempt status, moreover, the battle over civil rights has increasingly turned into a battle about whether discriminatory beliefs rooted in religion should be exempted from civil rights based on First Amendment freedom of expression.

This trend has peaked in the case of *303 Creative LLC v. Elenis*, which the U.S. Supreme Court decided in June 2023. The court ruled in favor of Lori Smith, the owner of a business creating websites for wedding announcements. Smith believes that homosexuality is sinful and announced plans to refuse service to LGBTQ people, asserting that forcing her to serve would amount to compelled speech in violation of the First Amendment. She asserted this despite the fact that Smith's business is in the state of Colorado, where there is a statute specifically forbidding discrimination based on gender or sexual orientation. In endorsing Smith's desire to discriminate against customers she doesn't like—while holding herself out as open for business per a license issued by the state—the Supreme Court dealt a major blow to the jurisprudence of unbiased public accommodation. Indeed her argument echoes the arguments of earlier civil rights cases in which segregation and refusals to serve Black people were rationalized based on religious belief: intermarriage was asserted to be "against God's law." Homosexuality was a religious "abomination." Jews and Indians were "heathens."

Smith essentially resurrected those old arguments by wrapping bigotry in the armor of religious freedom and aligning the assertion of freedom of religion with ultra-libertarian arguments about unbridled choice and personal preference. Civil rights laws and principles of public accommodation had come a long way since the 1960s; but in *303 Elenis*, the current Supreme Court failed to respect the line of reasoning that regards a business license as a grant *contingent* upon service to all members of the public without invidious discrimination. Instead it prioritized religion as a value greater than almost all others, allowing "freedom of speech or expression"—religious or otherwise—to be weaponized by the compression of constitutional ethics into a model of private and wholly individualized "choice."

This approach paves the way for the very notion of public accommodation to be fragmented into little zones of exclusionary prejudice. But for the increasingly fragile protections of the Civil Rights Act, it paves a path back to those little signs in the windows of restaurants announcing whole ranges of refusals: refusals to allow entry, service, bathrooms, or water fountains to Jews, Muslims, Mexicans, Blacks, "colored," Irish, "homosexuals," Chinese, Japanese, interracial couples, "cripples," and the blind.[11] That is my concern in all that follows. We have been this way before.

10

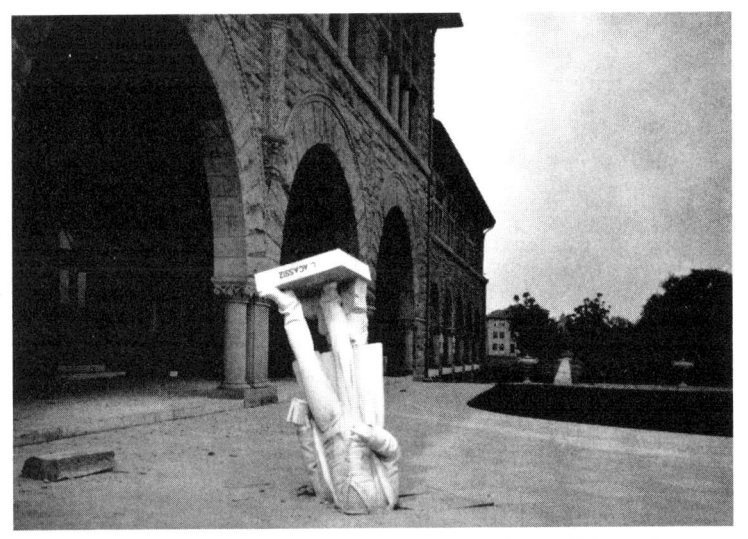

Proxy Wars

Louis Agassiz's statue at Stanford Universoty, California, having fallen to the ground after the San Francisco earthquake of 1906

Wikimedia Commons

There are many absurd assumptions about embodied Black difference abroad in our land: "They" can't swim because their bodies don't float. "They" can jump higher thanks to an extra muscle in their legs. The imagined Black body has a smaller brain, a bigger butt, a longer penis, saltier blood, wider feet, extra genes for aggression, thicker skin. Nor is this just history. Many dangerously unscientific beliefs about racial difference are baked into present-day pharmaceutical titrations and point-based algorithmic calculations, altering diagnoses of everything from incidence of skin cancer to diabetes to likelihood of osteoporosis to tolerance for pain.

Thus I greeted with great suspicion the news that, early in the pandemic, a Trump-era federal committee advising the Centers for Disease Control and Prevention was reported to have been considering who should be at the head of the line for any vaccine (then yet to be) developed for COVID-19; and that one idea being floated was whether those identified as Black and Latinx should be prioritized as distinguishably COVID-19-vulnerable populations. The idea was not implemented in the end. And when vaccines became widely available shortly thereafter, the problem was treated as moot. But it was disturbing that race was so unquestioningly deployed as a cipher for biological difference. The wrongheadedness of this exceeds concern about COVID-19. Given an increasingly crowded and overheating world, we are certain to face other deadly pandemics, sooner rather than later. We need to be absolutely clear in our ability to challenge the ethics of race-based medical allotments; we need to be able to understand and articulate why racial disparity in health outcome is not about biological difference.

There's no question that people of color were and are dying of COVID-19 (and a host of other diseases) at disproportionately unholy rates. In midsummer 2020, the age-adjusted data analyzed by the American Public Media Research Lab indicated that the widest disparities in American deaths afflicted Black, indigenous, and Latinx populations. Black mortality rates from COVID were from 2.3 to 3.7 times greater than those for whites. Indigenous rates are as much as 3.5 times higher, and those of Latinx people, two to three times higher.[1] When broken down by county, the death rate for predominantly Black counties was six times that of predominantly white counties. Indeed, all racial groups marked as minorities in America—including Asians, Latinos, and Pacific Islanders—are more likely than whites to die from COVID-19.[2] And the true picture may actually be much worse: during the worst of the crisis, the CDC had been weighting its calculations in ways that omitted geographies that have few-to-zero cases—which, coincidentally, just happened to be largely white areas. According to an article in the *Journal of the American Medical Association*, this weighted counting "understates COVID-19 mortality among Black, Latinx, and Asian individuals and overstates the burden among White individuals."[3]

The problem with assigning vaccine eligibility by race or ethnicity is the use of those political and social constructs as proxies for all the prejudices and vexed material conditions that make raced bodies more susceptible to begin with. In effect, it turns race into a signifier of innate disease propensity and physical disability. One may wonder why minorities' lower survival rates could not be more accurately described by referring to homelessness, dense housing, lack of health insurance, inadequate food supplies, and exposure to environmental toxins in the ghettoized geographies which have become such petri dishes of contagion.

This is not to suggest that discrimination suffered by Black and brown people is simply about class. In a nation shadowed by eugenic intuitions about "useless eaters" whose lives are deemed "not worth living," race is its own risk. American prejudices about color and race are rooted in powerful, long-term traditions of anti-miscegenation and untouchability: the propinquity of dark bodies—sometimes even so much as eye contact—incites anxiety and a fear of social contamination. Even to doctors, color can be an unacknowledged source of revulsion if they have grown up in all-white environments. It can operate affectively and aversively, like stigmatizing witchery. It's understandable why head-of-the-line vaccinations might be attractive to some, if only as a devil's bargain offering access to a resource perceived as otherwise inaccessible to Blacks and Latinx. But this is not just about head-of-the-line policies regarding a crisis whose crest seems now behind us. It is about managing scarce resources in dealing with any deadly contagious disease.

We must avoid building public health architectures that use race or ethnicity as the equivalent of innate, biological vulnerability—or, for that matter, invulnerability. In a stressed and overpopulated world, we must not facilitate what is already a competition over resources turning into an unseemly competition over "blood."

It is insidious to think of "race" as proxy for blood rather than the ambiguities of culture. Race cannot be determined with precision instruments: Is it how you look? Who you grew up with? The color of your eyes? Would ethnicity be determined by your name? Your neighborhood? Could contemporary assignments of race end up being an economic boondoggle for sketchy DNA testing companies? The simple fact is that looking at someone's color or social "place" and presuming all sorts of medical, criminological, and genetic predispositions is unscientific. By the same token, looking at a genetic variation and naming it after a more capacious, capricious, and/or unstable category like "Hispanic" or "Native American" is to write linguistic or cultural grouping onto genes.

This is precisely how 23andMe and other ancestry-tracking or direct-to-consumer companies seem to be rewriting race as biological. Some geneticists or biologists are thoughtlessly mapping all the social baggage of race onto the genome. It might not sell as well to those who are looking for romantic reconnection with lost "roots," but it would be a lot safer and saner and more scientific to use an entirely new or different symbolic vocabulary to mark allelic or haplotype groupings.

To reinscribe the convoluted, shape-shifting social baggage of racial division onto our biology actually creates a new golem, a doppelgänger of what we have historically thought of as race but a version that marks difference even more efficiently and insidiously than its older instantiations.

As far as we know, all humans are vulnerable to COVID-19—it was a pathogen new to our species. To assign race as causal in its spread is a category mistake. Even where certain diseases actually do cluster within particular populations, it is a mistake to describe such clusters as racial. Conditions such as enzyme deficiencies, tolerance for altitude, the ability to metabolize certain proteins or construct nucleic acids, and the susceptibility to certain diseases are distributed throughout our species. Humans are prone to a whole range of diseases we often delude ourselves into thinking of as the property of "only" particular ethnicities or races, such as Tay-Sachs among descendants of Ashkenazi Jews; Kawasaki disease as having a somewhat higher frequency among Japanese descendants; or sickle-cell anemia, often misleadingly called a "Black" disease rather than an equatorial or malaria-related disease; skin cancer, which I once heard a television doctor describe as something Black people "never" have to worry about. I guess he's never heard of Bob Marley.

All this shows that even high aggregations of frequency are no substitute for actual diagnoses. Mere correlation is not the same as cause and effect, yet epidemiological calculations are too frequently used as proxies for individual diagnoses, such as osteoporosis. For example, websites such as Medscape offer a vast menu of calculators designed to assign risk—including one to assign race in order to calculate one's risk of breaking a bone.[4] However, while less melanin (or lighter skin) is correlated with higher risk of osteoporosis, racial identity is not biologically revealing of melanin (or diet or exercise, also indicators of risk); race is a political designation, whose parameters vary from nation to nation and culture to culture. Those who are assigned whiteness can run a gamut of skin tones, and among those perceived as Black, there is a palette as broadly varied as humanity itself. A very light-skinned "Black" American might be as prone to osteoporosis as a blonde woman from Norway.

Moreover, even the very question of race is not one that is asked universally, but mainly in culturally freighted settings. The website FRAX, an internationally used fracture risk assessment calculator formulated at the University of Sheffield in the United Kingdom, has a calculator specifically for "USA use only," which distinguishes risk for "US (Caucasian)" from risk for "Black," "Hispanic," or "Asian."[5] Indeed, FRAX uses a "Calculation Tool" whose algorithm seems to conflate biological propensity with national identity. Indeed only four countries in FRAX's global index break national identity into separately calculated racialized subgroups: China (Chinese and Hong Kongers); Singapore (Chinese, Malay, Indian); and South Africa (African, Coloured, Indian, White). By the same racialized logic, Israel is listed under Europe, while its surrounding geography including Palestine, Syria, Saudi Arabia, Jordan, and Egypt are listed under Middle East and Africa.

It is impossible to know what distinctions are being made, what differences in dosages might be dictated by these political groupings. Even hypothesizing distinctly local forms of osteoporotic clustering, is there really a calculated distinction between "Caucasian" in the United States and "White" in South Africa? And if so, what is the measure of that calculation? My differentiated "Black" body in the United States would be calculated as just plain "Canadian" if I hopped across the border. That makes even less sense medically than it does politically. This data seems as though it's been divided up in ways that assume difference. The decision makers engineering FRAX's imposed metrics seem committed to an idea that national identity is a transparent cipher, and just "naturally" reflective of inherent biological difference.

To push the point just a little more, I am a woman of "a certain age," and doctors routinely use those two metrics—age and sex—as triggers for testing women over the age of sixty for osteopenia or osteoporosis. Thus, when I was given a routine bone scan recently, the results that came back to a computer on my doctor's desk were supposed to figure out whether I might need medication, using my individual data and predictive algorithms. The doctor sat behind his computer screen for a very long time. Finally, his head emerged from around the rim of the screen. He cleared his throat, and mumbled that the machine couldn't do the calculation, "probably because you're Black." Annoyed but undaunted, I told him just to sabotage that machine by telling it I was white. Based on that simple switch of identity alone, the system promptly presented me with a slew of additional questions: like whether I'd ever broken a bone, if so at what age, whether I showed signs of rheumatoid arthritis, and most urgently, whether there was osteoporosis in my family, especially my mother.

The fact that the machine would not have asked me any of that if I had been categorized as Black was machine bias of a profound and profoundly interesting sort. Indeed, although the machine apparently had categorized my Blackness as "self-identified," no one asked me about my heritage. Clearly some administrator or nurse had checked the box based on how purportedly and persistently "self-evident" or "obvious" race is thought to be within the American cultural context. The infinite spectrum of melanin inheritance is thus reductively "seen" as an either-or. In addition, the authority of my well-trained doctor, a human expert, was superseded by the narrow closed-loop small-mindedness of a black box containing only the pathways programmed by a nonmedical computer scientist who was apparently socialized to think about race as binary and blinding. The deference my doctor accorded the machine—and the deference most of us accord algorithms—dislocates particularized human expertise. Black-box medicine may be great at identifying and assessing broad patterns, but when it comes to the peculiarly complex intricacies of individual bodies in a nation of extraordinarily mixed and diasporic heritage, that deference to the machine can end up treating probabilities as though they were certainties or absolutes. In or out; all or nothing.

Thus, varying organic presentations of disease, as well as adaptations to varying ecological conditions (like famine, altitude, or inbreeding), are best thought of as precisely that: *variations* on a common human theme. And yet, to this day, many American medical schools teach that African Americans have greater muscle mass than whites. This is a fiction that dates to slavery, yet it informs how kidney disease is treated, for creatinine levels are used to measure kidney function, and greater muscularity can increase the release of creatinine in blood. But rather than assessing individual patients' actual muscle mass, most hospitals rely on an algorithm that automatically lowers Black patients' scores, thus delaying treatment in some instances by making all Black people appear healthier than they may be.[6]

Similarly, a test developed and endorsed by the American Heart Association weighs race in determining risk of heart failure. The algorithm automatically assigns three extra points to any "nonblack" patient; the higher the score, the greater the likelihood of being referred to a cardiology unit, yet there is no rationale for making Blackness a lesser risk factor in heart disease, and the AHA provides no reason.[7] Needless to say, Black and Latinx patients with the same symptoms as their white counterparts end up being referred for specialized care much less often. Underserviced, too many Black patients go unnoticed till they are at death's door with "sudden" or "aggressive" versions of common diseases. With endless irony, that is when those neglected bodies may become exceptionalized embodiments of "genetic difference." Medical historians, including Harriet Washington, Dorothy Roberts, Lundy Braun, Troy Duster, Jonathan Kahn, and Evelynn Hammonds have been complaining about such stereotypes and biases for decades, but perhaps it has taken the convergence of #BlackLivesMatter, a global health crisis, and a diverse new generation of outspoken medical personnel for this topic to have finally been taken seriously.[8]

I mention these stereotypes in order to ponder the medical consequence of such epistemic foolishness at a moment when COVID-19's disparate toll on Black and brown bodies has directed much attention to "underlying conditions." Careful commentators will point out that underlying conditions are not the same as innate predisposition; there is no known human immunity to this coronavirus. While age and illness may diminish our immune system's response to any pathogen, that greater susceptibility is merely a probability indicative of neither any human predisposition nor any natural immunity. Our universal susceptibility to it is underscored precisely by the virus's being "novel." It bears repeating that underlying conditions like rates of stress, diabetes, asthma, crowded living conditions, and overrepresentation in risky jobs are factors directly accounting for greater intensity of affliction. We know this—it is not a mystery.

Given this, attention to the fate of people of color is both overdue and double-edged: it highlights inequities but also risks reinforcing them as innate. For example, if the U.S. rates of infection are wildly off the charts compared to other nations, we do not generally blame it on the innate conditions of a peculiarly "American" biology; we know these numbers are the product of poor policy decisions. Just so, disproportionate deaths among communities of color must not be attributed to an imagined separateness of "African American"!

Amid a welter of misguided fantasies about "subspecies," "bad blood," and "dissolute traits," we forget at our peril that the trauma and social factors disproportionately affecting people of color are also driving death rates among whites—if not to the same degree. Trap white people in crowded, poisoned, impoverished contexts, and *they* die too.

Resurgent proposals to use race or ethnicity as a marker of disease vulnerability are appealing for their lifesaving potential when confined to the context of vaccine prioritization. But it remains to be seen how race is intersecting with vulnerability for purposes of triage in hospital settings. COVID-19 is capable of reducing us all to frail, wheezing, nonessential, bare bodies. When we arrive at the emergency room, we are delivered as mere bags of bones among so many "burdening" the health care system. Anonymously quarantined in isolated wards, not visibly being marked as a uniquely beloved soul with dear family and networks of friends is bad enough without having race deployed as an additional cipher for poor outcome. With a shortage of ICU beds, such a cipher is increasingly algorithmically weighted as well, for algorithms are more efficient than the Horae, and doctors are really quite busy these days.

Recognizing the risks of bias in such emergency circumstances, the Department of Health and Human Services' Office of Civil Rights issued a bulletin on March 28, 2020, restating a federal commitment to protecting "the equal dignity of every human life from ruthless utilitarianism." Under both the Americans with Disabilities Act and the Affordable Care Act, people "should not be denied medical care on the basis of stereotypes, assessments of quality of life, or judgments about a person's relative 'worth' based on the presence or absence of disabilities or age." The underlying concern is exemplified by the case of Michael Hickson, a Black quadriplegic whose COVID-19 care was withdrawn by St. David's South Austin Medical Center after a doctor told his wife: "His quality of life—he doesn't have much of one." His wife was recorded asking pointedly: "Because he's paralyzed with a brain injury, he doesn't have quality of life?" The doctor answered in the affirmative.[9]

The *New England Journal of Medicine* ran a number of articles about triage in the face of shortages of ventilators.[10] Here is one such take:

> Triage proceeds in three steps: 1. application of exclusion criteria, such as irreversible shock; 2. assessment of mortality risk using the Sequential Organ Failure Assessment (SOFA) score, to determine priority for initiating ventilation; and 3. repeat assessments over time, such that patients whose condition is not improving are removed from the ventilator to make it available for another patient.[11]

Number one covers the direst instances—crudely put, those who do not stand a chance. Number two, mortality risk, may encompass a lot of us who are older or who have disabilities or other preexisting conditions. And since there is overlap between long-term stress, environmental poisoning, poverty, lack of medical insurance, and such conditions, there is quite a perfect storm of collective mortality risk clustered by zip code and histories of real estate segregation. Number three, "repeat assessment" of whether to free life support for another patient is interpolated by availability of resources that will be in shorter and shorter supply as the numbers of sick and dying climb. Ideally, such assessment is supposed to be done by committee, in conversation with family members or surrogates, and done with consideration of a patient's Do Not Resuscitate orders.

But, in a pandemic or other emergency, decisions to withdraw care are frequently up to a single doctor, or resident, or perhaps a nurse. In other words, given mounting numbers, it will probably be up to a highly stressed, overworked, frightened, sleep-deprived human being who has no relation to you but the abstractions of your temperature, oxygenation rate, age, and whatever else that singular individual medical professional finds to read onto, into, or out of your body.

Discrimination against those with loosely defined disabilities is already quite common; the University of Washington Medical Center, for example, has argued for "weighing the survival of young, otherwise-healthy patients more heavily than that of older, chronically debilitated patients."[12] The reconfigured overlay of race, itself a debilitating, resource-consuming morbidity risk, worsens the situation. Disability rights advocates have worked hard to push these concerns to the front burner, urging Congress to ban triage based on "anticipated or demonstrated resource-intensity needs, the relative survival probabilities of patients deemed likely to benefit from medical treatment, and assessments of pre- or post-treatment quality of life."[13]

On July 22, 2020, the advocacy organization Disability Rights Texas filed a complaint with HHS against the North Central Texas Trauma Regional Advisory Council for its use of a rigid, point-based, algorithmic scoring system, which can automatically exclude from intensive care persons with a range of preexisting conditions and disabilities without resort to individual assessment.[14] Other states are beginning to reexamine their crisis rules in response to such concerns.

A way to avoid addressing the complexity of human identity, the reductivism of racial category is still far too common and far too misleading. Direct-to-consumer ancestry-tracking companies sell the promise of racialized "roots" and "identity" in often fallacious ways, and a broad swath of consumers fork out loads of cash to determine their genetic connection to fame, to fortune, and to name-brand-worthy ancestors. There has been a veritable surge of quasi-phrenological parlor games, so to speak.

That such testing can reveal ancestry based on broad migratory patterns over human history is not a surprise. Certain clusterings of genetic mutations over millennia occur more frequently among specific populations. Melanin concentration, for example, can reveal how one's ancestors adapted to more or less sunny climes. Nevertheless, there is no specific genetic marker that distinguishes one race from another. External differences—as in hair, skin color, and eye shape— are not linked to inner differences, no matter how strong the myths about skull size, extra leg muscles, or musical aptitude. I should think that this would all be abundantly clear by now, but there is remarkable persistence in reinscribing race onto the narrative of biological inheritance. This science is always pursued for only the noblest of reasons and the loftiest medical ideals, but if history has shown anything, it's that race is contradictory and unstable. Yet our linguistically embedded notions of race seem to be on the verge of transposing themselves yet again into a context where genetic percentages act as the ciphers for culture and status, as well as economic and political attributes.

I wonder, too, what becomes of liberalism itself when DNA, in addition to pinpointing how closely I'm related to Albert Einstein or whether I'm susceptible to a certain disease, can also recast my individual biological, medical, and mental quirks and differences-as-compared-to-others as "established" *in*equalities. This ability poses an interesting challenge to our presumptions of political equality, in that it is already beginning to spur policies that will privilege certain groups of people over others, if not as a matter of overt state policy, then as popular "privatized" eugenic "choice." Coming soon: preemptive quarantine or sterilization of those more prone to contracting certain diseases; preemptive detention of those prone to aggression; preemptive hiring; preemptive genetic alteration in favor of desired (meaning marketable rather than loved) qualities. A world of all sorts of well-meaning hierarchical mischief: whether the treasured allelomorph for blond hair or "gotcha" IQ numbers in a world where no one covets his neighbor's wife anymore, but only the market value of his neighbor's child's stratospheric SAT scores.

Why would one want to use DNA to track one's family history rather than excavate ancestral life lessons by more traditional narrative means? I suppose one obvious answer is that, for those of us who are descendants of slaves, it is precisely the lack of records other than our bodies—the traumatically aborted family narrative—that inspires the frantic pursuit of knowledge, the hunger for certainty, given generations of namelessness and rupture. At the same time, we must ponder: what are the limits of such biologized hindsight? How many graves must we dig up to complete ourselves? Is there not inevitable disappointment in the quest to know everything, to know absolutely?

Over the last few years, the American public-television-viewing public has been enjoying Henry Louis Gates Jr.'s series *Finding Your Roots*. They've been fascinating programs, especially from the perspective of history as a discipline. The series reveals the peculiar difficulties of tracking lines of descent through slavery—sales of human beings that acknowledged no family ties, the absence of last names, the absence of *first* names in some cases, and the necessity of consulting not just census records but also "the master's" property holdings for listings of possible relatives. The reconstruction of family history is like an archaeological dig, part intergenerational storytelling, part study of migratory patterns, part recovery of commercial transactions, and part science.

The science du jour is, of course, DNA testing, and here is where my interest tends to flag. On the one hand, DNA testing can be quite useful in establishing certain kinds of family relation. Gates's own test results showed that he has an Ashkenazi foremother, and that he has no relation to Samuel Brady, the white patriarch he'd grown up "knowing" as the man who impregnated his great-great-grandmother. His family lore had never hinted at what, in the *Wall Street Journal*, was playfully dubbed his "Yiddishe Mama."[15] By the same token, nothing had prepared him for Brady's *not* being his direct ancestor. Indeed, one of Gates's cousins remains adamant that the test must be wrong. If the test is right, he insists, there are two truths. One is the story he grew up with; the other is what the DNA says.

Somewhere in between what the DNA says and what shaped the family account is a gap that is something like an historical lie. A secret passing from Black to white? An act of assimilation or aspiration? A myth to hide some shame, some rape? A change of identity to escape to freedom? There is something very human, very moving about the repetition of family stories until they become epic rather than literal, about the burying of family secrets, the posturing of ancestors, the reinventions of migrants, the accommodations of raw ambition, the insulations from terrible shame. Such stories, I suppose, are distantly related to escapist manipulations; they might also be related to, but of a different order than, the magical thinking of mental patients or character-disordered people who claim to be the son of God, or a

Rockefeller, or heir to the throne of England. There is something so commonplace about the kinds of family mysteries that Gates's inquiries reveal—particularly in the American context. It is part of how many, many of our ancestors, regardless of where they came from, reinvented themselves in the New World. University of Pittsburgh law professor Jessie Allen describes the "magic" of legal remediation as follows: "What ought to have been prevails over the past."[16] Family stories ritualize the past in a very similar way. It is part of what Professor Robert Pollack, head of Columbia University's Center for the Study of Science and Religion, calls the "eschatology of repair."

If there is value to this kind of "emotional truth"—if I can be permitted that term—it is important not to confuse it with the sort of truth that DNA tells us. While DNA can undoubtedly pinpoint certain aspects of our ancestry, it does not make literal sense to say, as my mother once did, "You've got lawyers in your genes." Of course, she was speaking metaphorically, using the human genome as a metaphor for a pattern of socialization, a model to be attained—but genetic testing companies often seem to use race and nationality in ways in which the metaphor is not as transparent. White supremacists sometimes flatten continental origin into racial guarantee: a test finding of 90 percent "Northern European" becomes "I'm white." But there is no more an allele for "whiteness" than there is for "education." "White" is a malleable social designation with a freighted history and a loose geography. If Gates's Ashkenazi ancestors appeared before us today, they might be called white, but as Eastern or Southern Europeans coming to America a hundred years ago, they probably would not have been considered so.

I enjoy a weird genealogy of very old New England and the legacy of the slave trade. I was brought up in Boston at a time when the school system required not just reading but memorizing long declamatory polemics by Puritans, including Winthrop and Cotton and Danforth. My privileged but joyless education presented a world that had no norm but exceptionalism, no room for me but "difference" as a good thing, with no fair average of *its* own, never mind a room of *my* own. It left me with a peculiarly complex relation to my identity—a kind of learned exile despite being very rooted as an American. It's as though I were *also* a perpetually startled immigrant, if an immigrant to the familiar—placeless and unmoored even in a landscape of the intimately known.

Although I have expressed this latter feeling in terms of a personal trajectory, I suppose it's really about the power of an American narrative that places us all a little bit outside of ourselves, always a little bit beyond or behind the present moment, a design creating what Americanist Sacvan Bercovitch once called "a specific set of anticipations." I try to think about this in terms of symbolic forms of exclusion, inclusion, and exceptionalism, bringing them to the field of legal language, playing with them in the contexts of race, gender, bioethics, distributive justice, legal subjectivity, and personhood. I think of the peculiar covenantal appeal of Barack Obama's clever play with the conventions of the immigrant narrative, back during the 2008 election: Obama spoke of his immigrant father—not of a white European immigrant father who came to these shores in search of the American dream, but a Kenyan father, a Black immigrant, who came to these shores in search of heaven on earth. And his "single mother" wasn't the instant present-day stereotype of must-be-a-Black-woman, but was instead an unconventional *white* single mother, a self-searching multilingual anthropologist.

This calculated, unsettling reorganization of racial tropes played havoc with political and media expectations, and—for at least a little while—there was a grace period of suspended stereotypification as Obama inscribed himself within a very mainstream narrative trajectory of political candidacy. People just didn't know what to make of him; the finest example of such hand-wringing was then senator Joe Biden's amazement that Obama was just so "clean and articulate." It's hard to remember that tremulous moment of suspended judgment for what it was, because it so quickly evaporated; ultimately, Obama was not just exoticized but rendered so *familiarly alien* that even his birth certificate hasn't yet completely resolved the issue in some minds.

In years past, I have co-taught a seminar called Human Identity, DNA, and the Scientific Revolution, which was offered not just to law students but to graduate students from medicine, biology, journalism, and elsewhere and was part of Columbia University's core curriculum for selected college seniors. I co-taught it with three other professors: a biologist, a psychiatrist, and a philosopher/ethicist. One of the things that we were constantly working around was our very different senses of reference. Just take the word *nature*. It was a cellular reference to the biologist; it was a behavioral or chemical/pharmacological reference to the psychiatrist; to our philosopher, it invoked a moral ordering based in religious codes of natural law, like Vatican law. As a lawyer, I heard it as a normative social descriptor.

Or the word *human*. To the biologist it was an evolutionary category. To the psychiatrist, it was a fluid set of behaviors and intelligences that are not necessarily limited by the ability to mate as a species and could include tool makers and language users like parrots, apes, dolphins, elephants, and octopi. To the philosopher, *human* described a frailty. And to me, as a lawyer, it was a status that invoked a set of principles and sometimes rights that are derived largely from conventions premised on the notion of dignity.

In American law, the *human* is actually less important than the *person*. A *person* is an entity—biologically alive or imaginary, fictive or dead, sometimes human but not necessarily—to whom certain kinds of legal protections are owed. Hence, corporations, municipalities, and universities can be persons in that they can sue and be sued. They have standing and protection and recognition in our judicial and political system.

Therefore, when one of our law students wanted to write a paper about how dolphins should be extended personhood for purposes of bringing suits to protect their habitat and right to exist, our biologist was utterly confounded at first: his response was that dolphins aren't human. But in U.S. law, humans are not the only persons. The conversation grew only more heated and complex when one of our students opined that babies born with certain forms of encephalopathy that limit intellectual capacity might not be considered "human." That, in turn, opened a door to thinking about how scientists, academics, researchers, and doctors imagine the power of genetics. From that time on, I have asked my students to draw a cartoon depicting how they imagine the DNA in their own bodies. And no matter how sophisticated their scientific backgrounds, what they draw is almost relentlessly premodern:

Sometimes it's a set of little drones circulating just beneath the skin. Sometimes it's a little womb in the stomach, with a fully formed self, curled in a fetal position. Or it's a tiny scroll in a gold box just behind the thorax. (That's my favorite.) Or it's a mini-brain with a little engine that's churning all the time. Or a biological Torah in the Ark of the body. Or it's a homunculus in the alchemists' oven.

In the end, I urge them to fold up that piece of paper and set those romantic preconceptions aside. It behooves us all to be less romantic about what all this DNA swabbing reveals. I worry about the craving to "go back to Africa," or to "connect with our Italian-ness" or to feel as if new doors have been opened if one has an Asian ancestor. The craving, the connection, the newness of those doors is in our heads, not in our mitochondria. It is the process of superimposing the identities with which we were raised upon the culturally embedded, socially constructed imaginings about "the Other" we just almost might be. The fabulous nature of what is imagined can be liberating, invigorating—but it is fable. If we read that story into the eternity of our bloodlines, if we biologize our history, we will forever be less than we could be. Moreover, it will mark those who do not live up to that fantasy as "damaged goods" in a market for perfection. It is disturbing that so much cultural energy is spent assessing bodies for their utility rather than allowing them the comfort and acceptance we sometimes more easily extend to dogs and cats. We are often quite cruel to our fellow human beings, even our offspring.

For the last several years of my classes in bioethics, I've pondered the policy implications of the case of Ashley X, the "pillow angel."[17] Ashley was born with a debilitating form of encephalopathy that caused her brain to stop developing at about the age of three months. She is sensate, she smiles, she seems at times to recognize her family members and to enjoy music. But she can barely move on her own and will never learn to speak. When she was six, Ashley's parents contracted with Seattle Children's Hospital and subjected her body to a series of interventions ostensibly designed to keep her small, easy to lift and thus less prone to bedsores, and to render her permanently childlike.

To these ends, her breast buds were removed, in part because of a family history of breast cancer but, more immediately, to accommodate the harness straps that hold her upright. According to her parents' blog, "developed breasts . . . would only be a source of discomfort to her."[18] Her appendix was removed because, were she to get appendicitis, it was feared she would not be able to communicate her distress. She was given sufficiently high doses of estrogen to ensure that her growth plates would close, limiting her height. Estrogen at such doses carries other risks, most significant an increase in the incidence of blood clots, but her parents felt that being able to easily lift her outweighed that possible detriment. Her uterus, too, was removed, to spare her the pain of menstrual cramps "or pregnancy in the event of rape."

One of the more remarkable aspects of this case is that these surgeries were done without ever appointing a guardian ad litem for Ashley. No one within the hospital or its ethics board stopped to consider that it is illegal in all fifty states to sterilize a minor without such oversight.

While parents are assumed to have the best interests of their children in mind and to be able to consent on their behalf for routine medical procedures, this situation was hardly routine. Moreover, it conflated the interests of the parents as understandably burdened caretakers with the interests of Ashley who, for all her cognitive deficits, was not incapable of feeling pain. Indeed, who of us, with full capacity to consent, would undergo the painful invasiveness of a full hysterectomy just to prevent cramps or as a prophylactic against rape's violations? Why then should it be permitted in the case of someone who has no capacity to protest? Even assuming a life at the hands of sexual predators were so predestined a fate, why not birth control pills?

I believe that the outcome in this case was also wrong as a matter of ethics and public policy. There was, in the national debate about this case, a popular consensus that the parents were well motivated, so who are the rest of us to judge? That sentiment is expressed quite loftily in Princeton philosopher Peter Singer's *New York Times* op-ed: "She is precious not so much for what she is, but because her parents and siblings love her and care about her."[19] That general sentiment was expressed more crudely in an anonymous online posting to the disability rights organization FRIDA ("I think your group is a pain in the neck . . . if and when something happens to the caregiver, who will take care of the disabled person . . . your group or the state who really does not give a hoot.")

I do not question either how much Ashley's parents love their daughter or how overwhelming their responsibilities must be. I do, however, fault the hospital establishment for allowing these surgeries to happen—and to happen informally, without due process. In essence, the hospital allowed ethical questions about Ashley's long-term care and comfort to be privatized by deferring so unquestioningly to her parents' posited love. The hospital created an extreme presumption in favor of (often cash-strapped) caretakers that was heedless of medical necessity. Given a presumption premised on "love" rather than medical imperative, why not remove all her teeth to spare her the pain of cavities? Why not excise her fingernails to spare her the pain of accidentally scratching herself? Why not remove one of her healthy kidneys and donate it? That might make her and the world a little lighter. If I'm not the one who loves her, who am I to judge? That facile shrug allows us to ignore that Ashley's body was not altered to correct any physical need of her own but to address tenuous suppositions about long-term social pressures: she'd be more included in family events, she'd be less attractive to rapists (if not child molesters), she'd be more portable for the convenience of caretakers. Real medical benefits, such as lessened risks of cancers or appendicitis, were entirely speculative. (Indeed the hormones used to fuse her bone plates potentially increase her risk of cancer.)

Ashley's was the first such operation, but not the last: other children born with encephalopathy have been subjected to what is now known as the Ashley treatment. Much of the public debate has tended to dismiss regulatory oversight as some kind of invasion of privacy. But as medical ethicist Harriet Washington points out in her book *Medical Apartheid*, the very notion of privacy is inflected by the aesthetics of gender and race and class.[20] Ashley is—and now always will be—"cute," "little," and "a white girl," as some bloggers bluntly put it.[21] This embodiment evokes a very particular social response. It is harder to imagine doctors so compliantly agreeing to castrate a boy, say, in order to allow his wheelchair harness to fit better. Similarly, I wonder if a poor Black child would have been so easily romanticized as a "pillow angel."

The glib libertarianism of "Who are you to judge?" masks not only these inequalities of social response but also our failure to grapple with the woeful state of a health care system that leaves all Americans, even middle-class families like Ashley's, so burdened. We are the wealthiest nation on earth, yet we cannot find the resources to provide the common medical devices that would have better enabled

Ashley's family to care for her, unaltered, in their home: a simple hoist, mattresses that prevent bedsores, the assistance of home health care workers. Ashley's parents apparently felt driven to such lengths because they did not wish to institutionalize her as she grew older, bigger, more cumbersome. They feared her institutionalization with good reason, that fear reflecting but a fraction of the anxiety generated by our public health crisis.

If we reimagined Ashley's humanity as something larger than a private burden to be borne by a single family, we might align her debilitation with that of people with Alzheimer's disease or veterans whose bodies or minds have been shattered by war. Perhaps then the public health issues would be a bit more obvious. Perhaps then we might not turn so quickly to carving up the body as response to the scandalous deficiencies of our public hospital system, and the scandalous costs of our private one. Unlike Ashley, these men and women cannot be surgically miniaturized or pixied up with heavenly pet-name metaphors. They are full-grown, complex, their bodies heavy with sorrow, with need. Perhaps it is they who will provoke a collective reexamination—a call to judgment—of our polity's obligations to broader notions of human dignity.

Nor is this just about health per se. Remember that, cognitive limitations notwithstanding, Ashley's body was otherwise developmentally healthy. Our commitment to equal valuation of life is sorely tested by such examples of cost-benefit as human metric. I was pressed to think hard about this by a German ethicist: when I told her about the Ashley treatment, she described it as a "clear case of mutilation," and an attitude that sees disability—including economic disability—as a social burden and an unaffordable drain. She recited the history of Germany's period of economic devastation following World War I, just before the full-scale grip of Nazi rule in Germany. Hospitals became overwhelmed. Children with birth defects became an economic burden. The status of poverty slowly became subsumed to eugenic and germophobic legal stances on behalf of the body politic. "Mercy killing" of "useless eaters" gradually became labeled as "therapy." Hospitals and mental institutions quietly initiated more systematized bureaucracies of killing: children deemed "unsustainable" were marked for execution by a plus sign on their paperwork, their ultimate destiny identified as "disinfection," "cleaning," and "treatment." This was justified by the fascistic state of mind that psychiatrist Robert Jay Lifton calls "therapeutic survival"[22] or "the paradox of a 'killing self' being created on behalf of what one perceives as one's own healing or survival."[23] This, in turn metastasized into the mechanics of mass murder we know as the Final Solution.

This may seem an extreme comparison, a leap too far in the context of Ashley's situation. But I ponder nonetheless: perhaps it might serve as a thought exercise when paired with Dan Patrick's and Glenn Beck's conviction in the context of COVID that some human life might be too costly if it "kills the economy." I offer it here not to be tendentious, but only to highlight the slow, hypnotically encroaching cultural violence that can occur when the *nation's* body is insistently prioritized over the stricken human body.

We see all manner of emotionally wrenching legal messes in the cases of cognitive disability that hovers on the edge of mortality, not merely consciousness. In one extreme instance, the state of Texas tried to keep Marlise Muñoz, a deceased woman, on life support in order to sustain her fourteen-week-old fetus—this despite clear developmental injury and unsustainability of the fetus. Texas law provided that "A person may not withdraw or withhold life-sustaining treatment under this subchapter from a pregnant patient."[24] But Muñoz was not a "patient" any longer when her husband sued to have her removed from life support. She had already passed away from a massive brain hemorrhage, and her fetus had already suffered significant oxygen deprivation. While her husband ultimately won the injunction, the application of the law to a corpse was dependent upon an odd form of legal fictionalizing that literally deadened the mammalian interdependency of gestational processes. One must wonder if the Texas hospital that pressed its argument for the forcible extraction of use-value from Marlise Muñoz's body, ostensibly in order to bring her fetus to term, might have then gone on to handle that child's developmental problems with the same spirit of efficiently utilitarian surgical dispatch that Ashley met.

In any event, I have often wondered why the administration at Seattle Children's was so woefully inattentive to the propriety of seeking a hearing before performing radically experimental surgeries that included sterilization. My instinct is that philosophers like Nikolas Rose are quite right to point out that we have increasingly displaced the do-no-harm care ethic of "doctor-patient" with the choice-driven ethic of "service provider–consumer preference."[25] Consider the cases of parents who "gift" their teenage daughters with nose jobs or breast enhancement; or the family who adopted a baby girl from China, and then subjected her to plastic surgery in order to "westernize" her eyes.[26] The pervasive availability of elective plastic surgery is just one example of how issues of social stigma have been diverted by treating them as matters of contract. This habit of thought has shifted our attention in quiet but powerful ways away from the hard political work of maintaining our right to exist in the world without having to disguise, apologize, or suffer for our raced, gendered, or nonnormative bodies.

In the United States, we think of ourselves as "inalienably righted." Yet when gender, race, and class play against one another as they do in each of these stories, one sees demonstrated a tension between contract's sloshy alienations and the Constitution. This points to the ethical work to be done: those still uninterrogated forms of proprietary exploitation, of bodies, of identity, and ultimately of citizenship. Most pressingly, how do we account for nonnormativity and disabilities of all sorts, or for the silence of those who have no voice, or whose voices have become untranslatable? How do we—or do we at all—ventriloquize their desires, imagine their needs, try to compensate for what we perceive as their deficits?

This conundrum takes me to a very different context. I turn inward, thinking about a friend of mine, L., who suffers from early-onset Alzheimer's. I have known L. since we were teenagers, and my identification with her is strong and habitual; we have known each other well, I would say. Yet . . . even saying "I would say" in the context of Alzheimer's becomes permissive and self-licensing on my part, because she knows but doesn't know me from moment to moment. Her self-narration is fragmented, filled with gaps. In order to be a friend, I step back, live with the unknown; I teeter on the edge of understanding, live with the incoherent as norm. No longer a given, my knowledge of L. must yield to ignorance, and back again, a fluid kind of flipping. The uncertainty of her fugue requires that I yield and float. My friend is a cipher. My friend is indecipherable.

Once while I was driving her to a party, L. became quite fearful that "those things" were going to "fall on us." It took me some time to understand what she saw, what she "meant." It took me a while just to decipher that she was referring to the trees growing alongside the road. I couldn't tell whether she was afraid because the things she was seeing signaled fear of trees *as trees*—that they had dark spaces between and they might fall—or whether her fear was more from something like a view de novo. Like a child, like a baby seeing something for the first time, not knowing how to characterize or place it. I couldn't tell if the image with which she was struggling might be one of raw unfiltered sensation—stripes of darkness with floating green puffs on top. Thus envisioned, it might seem dangerously unstable. The mind would have nowhere to assign the vision.

She struggled so for the words with which to describe the trees. "The long narrow things," she said. "With the dark spaces in between. Those things over there. With the bushes on top."

"Tree trunks?" I finally asked. "Those are tree trunks."

"Yes," she said, tentatively, not entirely reassured.

Grappling with this complex world of miasmic confusion left me wondering about all the ways we forget *through* language. For example, my friend L. could have simply lost the word for tree—it might have been a "what's-its-name" to her.

Or maybe she became anxious because she had lost the cognitive word-bin for things "like" trees, a tree having become an altogether unfamiliar, nameless thing lacking a category. Words help sort and soothe through the intimacy of association. Words put what is unknown into cupboards labeled "known." Words are like nice little laundry hampers—the kind that segregate whites from colors from permanent press. Perhaps my friend L. was attempting to craft a personalized, but nonnormative, system of indication, as when she tried this: "Green clouds floating in a dark sky with skinny sticks stuck in the ground that might fall."

Or perhaps she was struggling with a deeper loss not just of words but of seeing: perhaps she couldn't apprehend discrete shapes as separate objects, but rather saw a blurry slush of a sensory-scape. Perhaps it was an impairment in distinguishing boundaries, an envisioning in which everything was part of everything, all just splotches of darkness and light. I wondered if she had lost the facility to disaggregate tree parts from an undifferentiated mass of visual input of color and light and dark and line and form. Perhaps she had lost the ability to pick out foreground from background, or near-green parts from sky parts from deep shadow parts from bark-brown parts.

Such departure through forgetting demands reflection upon the nature of human communion. How in the end do we deal with the inscrutability of others? Perhaps the best we can do is hold still and listen. It is so tempting to fashion others' silence into obituaries, with hubristic disregard and in one's own image. It is much too tempting to wallpaper another's illegibility with one's own narrative of tragedy or loss or survival or uplift. But surely such a situation demands an ethic that takes into account the ever changing responsibilities of relation, repair, oblivion, and death.

I return to my preoccupation: How might we ever heal loss with sufficient ritual that the mind can let go, freed from bitterness or desire for retribution? Then one can relinquish what scholar Svetlana Boym called "restorative nostalgia," which "thinks it's possible to go home again. It sets out to re-create the past precisely and impose it on the future."[27] Such restorative nostalgia is all the more problematic when that supposed past, that sense of home, is a Disney-fied reduction, when it leaves out any coexisting horrors that might complicate or underwrite that yearning for idyllic re-creations.

11

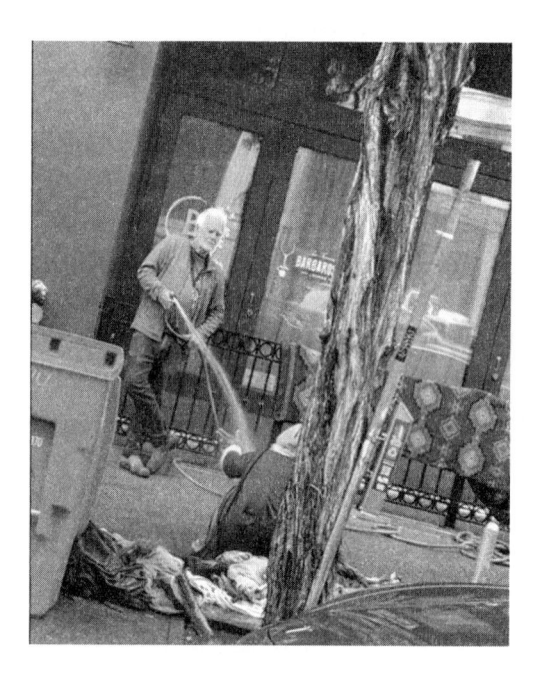

Dogsbody

In January 2023, the owner of an upscale art gallery in San Francisco, apparently channeling Bull Connor, used a hose to dislodge a homeless woman from sleeping in front of his business.[1] At around six a.m. on a very cold winter day, he used what was widely described as a "garden hose" to thoroughly soak the woman while shouting at her to move. It was a misnomer to refer to it as a "garden" hose. It was the kind of hose used in cities where there are precious few gardens—the hose that in urban environments is used like a broom, to spray the sidewalks first thing in the morning, to wash leaves, vomit, orange peels, MacDonald's wrappers, and dog poo into the gutter. A garbage-sweeping hose. The video—captured by an indignant deliveryman—surely contributed to the virality of this incident. It showed an aristocratic-looking white gallerist of considerable social position affecting an easy lean against a wrought iron fence, one leg crossed over the other, casually yet persistently hosing a mentally ill, distraught old Black lady as though she were a particularly sticky bit of sidewalk scum.

In subsequent interviews, the man's defense of his actions fell far south of rehabilitation. "I snapped," he admitted. But he did not feel the need to apologize further because he blamed the city for not solving what he framed as *his* problem: he explained that he had called the police many times before, attempting to get the woman transported somewhere else. No one took her out of his field of vision. So that morning he was unbearably stressed when she "belligerently" refused to move while "speaking in tongues."

He just didn't know what else to do: it was an attempted *kindness* to her, to call upon the gods of hypothermia.[2]

My thoughts turn to the homeless man who sets up camp on a sidewalk in the financial district of my city. He has a plastic cup and a handwritten cardboard sign, asking for contributions. The man also has a dog, a big lantern-jawed boxer mix. The pair is there every day, rain or shine, and there is usually some passerby engaged in conversation—always about the dog, and sometimes even *with* the dog. "Hello Doggie!" they begin brightly, before turning a gimlet eye upon the homeless man, demanding to know whether the dog has had his shots or whether the dog has adequate protection from the cold in winter, and whether the dog has been taken for regular visits with a vet. "*I'm* a vet," whispers the homeless man to that last, with no hint of irony. "I love my dog. I take good care of him."

Recently, I was traveling from Washington, DC, to Boston. I

settled in to wait at Gate J of Union Station with my knitting and a book of crossword puzzles. A woman dressed in the multiple layers of someone who has donned everything she owns sat down two seats away from me: she was wearing a linty black knit cap drawn over short dreadlocks, an oversize stained sweatshirt, and baggy maroon trousers. She carried several smudged and well-worn shopping bags that she arranged in a semicircle at her feet and began talking to them, commiserating about the terrible state of the world. Her tone was gentle, conversational, light. At first I thought she was speaking on a cell phone—there were polite pauses in what she said, moments of agreement and playfulness, seemingly rational responses to unheard questions—but in fact she was not.

She mourned the loss of democratic process in the Senate, the rise of mercenary armies and agribusiness, as well as the concentration of corporate power in the manufacture of butter and detergents ("It looks like there are a thousand brands on the shelves, but in fact they're all owned by one or two multinationals.") She feared the social consequences of the financial crisis: "Things that should protect our economy . . . the Robinson-Patman Act . . . they're so busy undoing, that that undoing will *be* our undoing."

Genius? Insanity? Either way, her observations threw me for a loop—they were illuminating, mesmerizing, shocking, dislocating. I dug my iPhone from my bag and googled the Robinson-Patman Act. In some other universe, I used to know what it said.

According to Foucault's *The Birth of the Clinic*, the "first structure provided by classificatory medicine is the flat surface of perpetual simultaneity."[3] As the tiny blue screen of my iPhone fluttered and winked to life in its search for meaning, I gazed about the waiting area of Gate J, Union Station. Nearly everyone was similarly engaged with their cyberspatial phylacteries, davening into thin air, entranced, uttering streams of words that echoed in the high-domed space like a turbulent waterfall. Unlike the woman next to me, however, they all seemed to be deploying visible blue-tooth devices or earplugs affixed to their heads, their eyes flat, inwardly transfixed.

Thirty-five years ago, I suppose, the place would have seemed like a ward at Bellevue. A well-dressed man across from me was enunciating loudly about having to reschedule a game of handball. A woman with a messily overstuffed briefcase had her head cocked like an eager spaniel's in order to keep her phone tucked in the hollow between shoulder and neck; she murmured over and over, "Uh-huh, . . . uh-huh, . . . uh-huh, . . . uh-huh," like a series of involuntary spasms. A college student in a porkpie hat congratulated a colleague upon his recent engagement and promised to throw him a bachelor party with lots of "juicy, big-lipped prostitutes, dude." A guy in a hoodie and mud-spattered Timberland boots was waxing lively about "some people" who don't want to "move their fat butts and work." Not on a cell phone was the exception—a wiry child of about ten with alarming, much-too-bright eyes, who darted around the benches, seeking "a dollar for food."

Thirty-five years ago, after all, it was still springtime in America. The thought of a political crisis as deep as ours crossed few minds outside the more perspicacious—some said paranoid—in the quadrants of academia and, of course, the perpetually redlined limits of inner cities. This day, the waiting room at Union Station was ablaze with the alternating semaphores of legitimacy, exhaustion, the absurd. My head spun with fatigue and the roaring heteroglossia. Next to me, the woman in the linty hat was telling the same story over and over: she moved so fluently among the disappointments of commerce, politics, law enforcement, and grammatical apocalypse ("You need to end that sentence with a question mark, young lady!"). I struggled to track the coherence in her constantly disrupted narrative.

An amiably demeanored security guard strolled by. He nudged at the woman's circle of bags with his shoe and told her to move along. She gathered her belongings with a great expenditure of crinkling rearrangement, the flow of her words never ceasing. There was a particularly intriguing riff about the police having killed her, followed by a soft, wise little laugh: "But you can't let your kin kill you either."

Then, still addressing the epistemic gatekeeper within, she offered shyly: "You are very well liked."

"Thanks," she responded brightly to herself, and shuffled off.

The District of Columbia has among the highest percentages of homelessness in the nation. African Americans, veterans, and the mentally ill are disproportionately represented among their ranks. When the pandemic began to level the playing fields of misfortune just a bit, non–African Americans, nonveterans and the certifiably sane struggled madly to distinguish themselves from the usual narratives of poverty: laziness, lack of qualifications, bad choice. A determined dis-identification with our preexisting populations of internally displaced edged into the national parlance, with a host of predictable resentments. The possibility that we, the broad collective of people, were sinking into a communal financial ooze was underestimated, rationalized instead as the fault of the ones who sank first. From Fox News to the blogosphere, such analysis focuses on blaming those on the bottom for being too heavy, weighing too much, and generally dragging the rest down.

In *Madness and Civilization*, Foucault wrote: "If we try to assign a value, in and of itself, outside its relations to the dream and with error, to classical unreason, we must understand it not as reason diseased, or as reason lost or alienated, but quite simply as *reason dazzled*." By the same token, the failure to see our common fate defines a dangerously bedazzling split between spirit and logic; between poetry and engineering; between the messiness of mercy and, ultimately, the orderliness of law.

Some days later, I was sharing a private shuttle ferrying a group of us to a gala dinner after a conference on fundraising and philanthropy. It was attended by a few of us public interest academics, but most of the international participants were the beneficiaries of both great wealth and generous spirits. They wanted to make the world a better place and were attending events like this in order to study how to allocate their assets. The shuttle bus pulled up to a stoplight. A homeless man stood at the intersection with a tattered cardboard sign upon which had been scrawled: Please help. Need money for food.

"Wow," said one of the more major donors in the group. "How sad! You just don't see that sort of thing in the United States." The donor is American—a good man, a nice man, whom I consider a pretty close friend. I prepared to say something snappily sardonic, tease him about not having gotten out of the house in the last twenty years. *Ever ride the subway?* I'd wanted to ask while shaking my head and rolling my eyes. At that moment in time, New York City's population included over seventy thousand unhoused people.[4] Murmurs of assent emerged from a number of the others on the bus, whom I knew less well. I bit my tongue. I felt literally out of my league. It took me a minute to realize that our experiences were different in what initially had seemed small but turned out to be profoundly substantial ways: These were good people who actually did *not* ride the subway. Who didn't walk the streets. Who helicoptered everywhere, from rooftop to rooftop. Their view of the world was sincerely limited by the efficiencies of their lifestyle.

But . . . still . . . these were also people who read newspapers. Who subscribed to the *New York Times*. Surely they would have read that approximately 16 percent of New York City residents live in poverty.[5] I suppose you can read about such things and still not have it register as the kind of desperation that results in standing on street corners begging for handouts. It's one thing to read about a man who tries to cope with only $5 a month left for food after paying for housing and transportation to his job. It's another to link that story to the apparition of bedraggled families rummaging through dumpsters.

I wanted to speak, to say "look up at the world." But I have been chided before by this group for speaking too harshly, for speaking as though I were engaged in class warfare. I do have a teacherly, preacherly tongue when I get going. What would I, who live in an ivory tower, know about it anyway? It's hard to tweak some of them about things like this because they are human and vulnerable and take it personally. And, again . . . w*hat do I know about it anyway?* We all want to be seen as innocent and forces for good in the world. We all have our pride.

It is a delicate matter to tell someone that you believe they have a blind spot about anything at all. We are all so human and vulnerable. We are all so easily dismembered. But persistent inattention to the dire crisis of homelessness hardens us, blinds us. The homeless, the unsheltered, people living on the periphery, are not only seen as "useless" but are increasingly treated as worse than useless, "bad for business." They are seen not merely as the sign of an unhealthy economy but, more troubling, their very existence becomes the *cause* of a sickening economy. This in turn seems to have rationalized treatment that is deadly: the intentional removal of public bathroom facilities; removal of the homeless themselves to remote and inhospitable locations in the desert; laws that fine or punish Good Samaritans for placing stores of water in the desert; intentionally caging migrants in cells so cold they became colloquially known as refrigerators or doghouses . . . for "dogs' bodies."

12

The Dispossessed

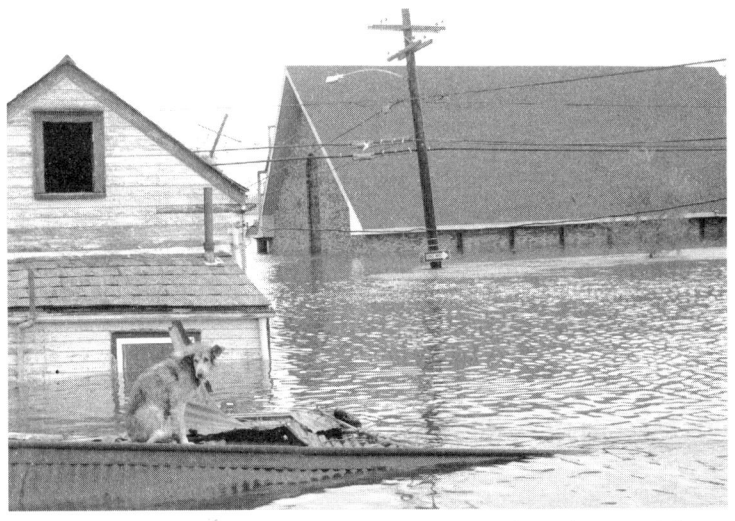

A dog sits stranded on a rooftop in the flooded Lower Ninth Ward in New Orleans, Louisiana on August 29, 2005. Hurricane Katrina slammed Louisiana as a category 4 storm, forcing levies to break and flooding much of New Orleans.

Photo by Marko Georgiev/Getty Images

One definition of trauma is that it is an injury so great that no words can capture or describe it. Faced with the insufficiency of language, the victim performs or experiences that horror over and over again, in the form of dreams or flashbacks or acting out. Hurricane Katrina was and continues to be an unparalleled trauma upon the body of American society. Many people have described it as the greatest natural disaster in our history, but there was little that was "natural" or inevitable about it. In the years hence, the violence of the storm has been exceeded many times over—in storms that have devastated Puerto Rico, the Bahamas, the Virgin Islands, and the Florida Keys. Around the world, of course, the force of ecological disasters has grown exponentially as carbon emissions have soared, as polar ice has melted, as the Amazon has been burned, as climate degradation has proceeded unchecked in any significant way.

However, the wound that Katrina left resulted from a complicated intersection of social forces that implicate much more than climate change alone: from the failure to heed many years' worth of warnings about the deteriorated condition of the levees to the failure to initiate mandatory evacuation proceedings well before the storm hit; from the corruption that rendered regional government so perpetually ineffectual to the corporate muggery that has left this richly endowed arable delta impoverished and poisoned; from the cruel and inhuman conditions in the Louisiana state penitentiary known as Angola to the school system that was and remains little more than a prison industrial complex itself.

Except as a matter of degree (or as a matter of pure size), all of this is familiar. Indeed, it is so entirely familiar that it practically seems predestined. Public and low-income housing razed to make way for corporate interests. Elderly left unattended on their deathbeds. Homeless children with more weapons than hope. A diaspora of broken families hunting for kin: Have you seen my mother? Have you seen my brother? This is a picture of my fiancée. . . .

The chilling ghostliness of such reiteration is not about what has already happened; ghosts are most frightening when they drift from memory to the visible present, then become the lens for our future. The horrors of Katrina form an ongoing narrative of national distress, of aimless migration, of homelessness, of exile. If the Puritan jeremiads envisioned our nation as a promised land, a new Canaan, a latter-day Jerusalem, our twenty-first-century jeremiad rewrites itself as paradise lost: as a tale of broken covenants, of much crying in the wilderness, of New Orleanians being swallowed by a sea of red ink, without trace, without mourning, without cultural memory.

Close on the heels of the hurricane came revelations of national patterns of predatory lending and our massive home foreclosure crisis. A bitter, confused, if thoroughly American narrative began to swirl: Doom is nigh, what a sucker you've been, and now no one's going to save you. . . . You didn't pack for eternal exile? Well it's your own dumb fault.

Homelessness rather than nudity is the great shame of the post-Edenic state. Against this backdrop, the peculiar locution of "homeland" "security" becomes a threatened terrain to be hunkered down inside but not lived within. The "homeland" is a Swiss cheese of unguarded portals, disposable trailer parks, promiscuous doorways, and floodgates that don't work—yet simultaneously and curiously devoid of real houses or real homes. In contrast, the simplicity of "home" becomes a site for nostalgia, the old country before famine, flood, or pogrom, an imaginary geography of tremendous contradiction, of ambivalence and flight, of (up)rootedness and romance, of magic and superstition.

This theme of the terrible sublimity of loss dominates our literary and political figurations, and unless addressed, or until healed, no doubt will continue to do so. It is the plotline of the evangelical works of Timothy LaHaye's *Left Behind* series,[1] of William Luther Pierce's *The Turner Diaries*,[2] as well as the tension in Toni Morrison's *Beloved* and Longfellow's *Evangeline*.[3] It runs through the babble on Fox News, in television dramas like *24*, in Samuel Huntington's book *Clash of Civilizations*,[4] and other doomsday political futurism. Loss shapes our domestic police practices and informs our global war on terror. It is echoed in far-right fears of "the great replacement," as well as in left-leaning legal suits like *Juliana v. United States*,[5] an attempt to frame children's rights to a pollution-free future as a demand that the federal government act more assertively in its role as a public trustee of natural resources.

As right and left tussle, there's a certain schadenfreude to our increasingly desperate sense of futility, the frisson of a well-rehearsed nightmare, the creed, the screed, the Greek chorus, the litany of woe, the passion play whose dark moral law haunts us ceaselessly.

When I think about the human disaster that has unfolded in the wake of Hurricane Katrina, two moments stand out in my mind. The first is George W. Bush's press conference in Mississippi on September 2, 2005, during which he bounced uneasily from foot to foot as if he couldn't wait to get out of there, looking sullen and furrowed, observing with tense jocularity that then senator Trent Lott's house had been lost, too, and that "we" were going to rebuild him "a fantastic house" and that he, our president, was looking forward to rocking on the porch when that day came to pass.

The second moment was the now-famous interview with Homeland Security chief Michael Chertoff on National Public Radio. Media junkie that I am, I had the TV and the radio on at the same time. As pictures of the horrific conditions at the convention center, including the image of the body of that poor old woman who had passed away in her wheelchair, were being broadcast to the world, Chertoff was insisting that he had no knowledge of any extreme conditions or deaths at the center. "Our reporter has seen [it]," insisted the host. "I can't argue with you about what your reporter tells you," said Chertoff with snappish impatience.

I confess that I was filtering this horror through a very personal lens. It overlapped with the task of clearing out and selling the house I grew up in, in Massachusetts, the house my mother was born in, my grandmother's house, a house that had belonged to my family for almost a hundred years. My distress at having to give it up is confused with the scenes of Katrina's devastation that most of us—if not Chertoff—were witnessing. Against that appalling backdrop I found myself clinging to a sense of place, even though I was not truly or traumatically displaced. Mine was an African American family that owned a home in times when so few did.

I still think hard about this as I look at the continuing devastation of the Ninth Ward, an area that, before the storm, had more African American property owners than anyplace else in Louisiana. As I drove back and forth from the house I grew up in, carrying out pictures of my college graduation and my Latin notes from seventh grade, I heard a woman on the radio describe how jarring it was to see the media describe her neighborhood as one riven by poverty and desperation. She was about to get her MBA, her brother already had his MBA, their extended family owned nine homes there, they all had insurance, and they all owned cars in which they had fled for their lives. But it was the Ninth Ward; it was indeed being dubbed "poverty-stricken," "corrupt," "drug-ridden"; and politicians like Dennis Hastert were talking about bulldozing the entire area.

The Ninth Ward, Gentilly, and other Black neighborhoods haven't been entirely bulldozed in the years since. But despite all the talk about rights of return, the only thing that's happened since—at least in the way of publicly funded reconstitution—has been the planting of a few strips of grass in front of still-empty buildings. Millions of dollars have gone into setting up charter schools, particularly in the suburbs, and tens of millions have been spent on metal detectors for the few public schools remaining within the city limits. The budget for books, meanwhile has been infinitesimal.

And so I still think about what might have happened if I had not been engaged in the relatively leisurely process of packing up my memories but had been forced to run for my life. In particular, the documentation of people being "sorted" in the shelters should give us pause. The elderly were taken from their families, the sick from their caretakers, newborns from their mothers, and, because men were apparently segregated from women, husbands were taken from wives, mothers from sons. I heard one unidentified local authority on the radio saying that when people were evacuated to other states, they were not told where they were going, so as to make them less unruly. And there were accounts of white foreign nationals airlifted out "secretly" by National Guardsmen and warned not to go into the shelters because it was too dangerous for them. To some extent, this sorting and separation is what already happens in homeless shelters in many places around the country, and even more so with noncitizens in immigration detention centers. Hurricane Katrina merely made that reality, at least momentarily, impossible to repress.

The rationalization of such practices proceeds unchecked, however. The supposed logic of Katrina's evacuation procedures followed a template even more cruelly deployed years later in President Donald Trump's family separation policies imposed on migrants fleeing instability in Central America. A few days into the seething mess at the Convention Center, a sociologist named Betty Hearn Morrow opined on NPR that it was less traumatic for people in distress to be grouped by their own kind. "That's just human nature," said Morrow. Putting people into groups reinforces a sense of familiarity and security, so they should be relocated "according to their backgrounds." She gave an example of sorting people from Guatemala and Nicaragua and explained how that would help keep the peace—though she did not explain how separating Americans from Americans would do the same.

My ears pricked up at this take on civil society; I wondered what "kind" I might appear to be in an evacuation. My son, fifteen years old at that time, was six feet four inches tall. If we were fleeing without any identification, would anyone believe he was a child? Would we be put on separate buses to unknown compass points? Would I be herded off to the camp for over-the-hill law professors? And if that's too scary to contemplate, would it really becalm me with a sense of "familiarity" to be penned up and marched off with a group of other Black women of my "background"?

In the wake of Katrina, American cities formulated evacuation plans. According to then-mayor Michael Bloomberg, the City of New York had been divided into grids in case of catastrophe. People would be ordered from their homes, or taken by force if necessary, and marshaled along preset routes to reception centers, where they would be identified by Social Security number and then relocated. I want to be a good citizen, part of the orderliness of a well-managed response to disaster. But with the images of New Orleans in mind, why on earth would any of us stream willingly toward chaos? If it is true that families may be broken up as a means of crowd control, then perhaps just a little public discussion is in order. And if it is true that white foreign nationals are a higher priority than Black solid citizens, to what then do we pledge allegiance?

As for the homeland and its infinite insecurity, new categories of suspect profiles bubble forth. Race, ethnicity, religion, a fortiori—but the list churns on with up-to-the-minute brands of scoundrels like an endless ticker tape: Unusually clean-shaven men, men with long beards, people wearing heavy clothing or shoes with thick soles or big hats, women carrying large handbags, unknown deliverymen bearing oversize packages, kids with backpacks or violin cases, sweaty people, cool-as-a-sly-cucumber people, people with cameras, people praying aloud, people who blink too much or not enough, men with thick waists, women pretending to be pregnant, people who spend too much time in public libraries, men reeking of rosewater—on and on it goes. Most recently, we are to be on the lookout for the great masses of the unshaved, unwashed, and unperfumed, to wit, "vagrants who seem out of place"—an almost calculatedly redundant designation—for fear they might be terrorists posing as "homeless people, shoe-shiners, street vendors or street sweepers."

In our once celestial cities, whose denizens are now deemed dangerous, one hears calls for house-to-house searches, shoot-to-kill policies, and protection from "too many" civil rights. Debates rage about "political correctness" rather than whether this isn't beginning to look like martial law, or an effective immunization of police from discriminatory behavior, scattershot decision making as well as deadly mistake. LOOTERS WILL BE SHOT, read signs posted in New Orleans post-Katrina.

I ponder this global game of "gotcha." It is a traumatically insistent re-presentation of a violent past, as well as a prefiguration of devastations to come. With this endless looping, our civic domesticity becomes ever more embittered, tainted by the obsession with enemies among us whose voices speak like the ghost of Hamlet's father, whose shapes we profess to "know" instinctively and in defiance of fancy rituals of politeness, legal niceties, book learning, or empirical knowledge.

I spent a few days in New Orleans recently. Years after the hurricane (and others that follow, follow, follow), it is still a city in mourning, as riven as ever. In 2000, before Katrina, the population was 484,674; in the immediate wake of the hurricane, the population fell by more than half, so that in 2007, it was a mere 239,124.[6] An estimated 30 to 40 percent of the population never returned, most because they have not been able to; by 2020, the population was still only 383,827.[7] Landlords refused to accept out-of-state housing vouchers from renters trying to return. Rents soared because of the decreased housing stock. Yet the New Orleans City Council demolished virtually all the surviving stock of public housing—large brick-and-mortar buildings, all minimally damaged, lots of windows blown out but all eminently reparable if there had been anything like an intelligent will. The tenants were never even permitted to go back in and retrieve their belongings.[8]

Today, the Lower Ninth Ward is an eerily lush plain of overgrown sadness. Despite all the attention given to specific projects undertaken by architect Frank Gehry and actor Brad Pitt, the rebuilding has been sparse and terribly slow. Of the ward's fourteen thousand residents before the storm, fewer than five thousand remain today.[9]

Only a few hundred buildings were sufficiently renovated for actual occupancy. Foreclosure rates were, predictably, staggering. I visited the city a number of times in the wake of the hurricane, and one of the more intriguing embellishments upon the expansive devastation was the flutter of hundreds of little signs affixed to the remaining lampposts: Easy terms! Refinance with us! and Want to rebuild? No money down! Local newspapers were full of disturbingly gushy articles about Realtors who slavered over the historic row houses still standing in largely Black and poor areas. They saw the next SoHo! The new Chelsea!

To hasten the process of what one half calls gentrification and the other half feels as dispossession, the city passed an "anti-blight" ordinance. Little signs were planted in front of houses where only the walls remained. "Do you know where this owner is?" These signs pass as public notice: found owners are slapped with anti-blight fines. Failure to pay results in forfeiture of the land.

A year after Katrina, flooding caused levees to burst again, this time on the upper Mississippi, making mud of Cedar Rapids, Iowa. Radio commentator Rush Limbaugh (he used to be thought of as a "shock jock" but his legacy lives on as an American norm) snickered that the (largely white) residents there weren't "whining" about their condition like those noisy (implicitly Black) New Orleanians. Well, it's quiet in New Orleans now, a terrible brew of frustration beyond words and utter exhaustion. If it is just as quiet in the largely white floodplains of the upper Mississippi, we should not take that for a good thing in an economy as troubled as ours. The collapsed levees in Iowa and Missouri are signs of the same deeply broken infrastructure, even if the corruption that allowed it is not as visible, as cruel, or as racially inflected as in New Orleans.

American mobility depends upon the equity accumulated in its homes and the stability lent by reasonable rental stocks. The failure to make affordable housing a right has, in the long run of the last half century, hurt all Americans, leaving us with ravaged "inner cities" and strip-malled "havens" of suburban blight. As I experienced New Orleans while visiting in 2008, two models compete for our future, unfolding on the street. Model Number One: while walking in the Eighth and Ninth Wards, I saw scores of volunteers from all over North America, a rainbow coalition of mostly young people and college students, working for organizations like Habitat for Humanity. They were sweating in the broiling sun, hard at work, hammers in hand. Model Number Two: I overheard a conversation between two middle-aged men apparently touring the same area "for property deals." The first was wearing an Obama T-shirt. The second said amiably, "So, you're for Obama." No, replied the first man; he was "a liberal," but he hadn't decided yet. It turns out he was a speculator in sheep's clothing, just wearing the shirt to ingratiate himself with the natives—although *ingratiate* was not the word he used.

Poor us. The course we pursue may be politically disastrous, academically wrong, strategically flawed, statistically disproved—a cacophony of finger-pointing and calls to 911—but our narratives instruct us to be stubborn guardians of the faith. At our collective peril do we remain enchanted by homiletic hokum about sifting wheat from chaff.

Of course, New Orleans is just one vulgar iteration of an inner city being "rediscovered," "reclaimed," and "repossessed" by moneyed interests. But the manipulations by which that has been and is being accomplished in New Orleans have seemed particularly convoluted and cruel.

So here's an observation, about a subject I cannot yet translate into the domain of specific remediation. I offer it as . . . just a story, because the politics of what I am about to describe challenge me so profoundly. Indeed, my own involvement in it probably exemplifies a certain kind of well-meaning but troubling liberal paradox.

Recently, I traveled to New Orleans for an event that had been organized by an arts foundation I do some work for. I went as part of a convening of nonprofit arts organizations from all over the country. The whole event was part of an effort to support artists and artists' spaces in that city, so many having been devastated in the wake of the flooding.

One of the events I attended was a spoken-word presentation under a tent, set up in a vacant lot in the Eighth Ward. The performances were very varied—song recitals by children, excerpts from plays with modern dance solos, poetry slams, and lots of bluesy music. Eventually, one woman rose and performed a long prose poem about her husband's funeral. It was a lament for the passing of tradition. She had wanted a jazz band to accompany his casket through the streets, the way all the members of her family had always been taken home to rest. But since the flood, the city of New Orleans had imposed a fee of $5,000. It cost $5,000 to get a permit to play music in the streets nowadays, and she didn't have that money, so her husband had to be buried without the fullness of the mourning tradition with which she always lived and had expected.

At the end of her elaborately and eloquently detailed presentation of the pain she had experienced, seemingly magically, members of a neighborhood social aid and pleasure club materialized—dressed in feathers and sashes, bearing trombones, trumpets, and tubas. They mounted the stage and began to play. They surrounded the woman, and then, still playing, not a dirge but a joyful recessional, they proceeded down from the stage, sweeping the woman along with them, and they marched out onto the street. The entire audience from beneath the tent, followed them, dancing, sashaying, trotting along to the music.

I had never been part of a so-called second line and considered myself very lucky. People poured out of their houses to join the line. I merged with the crowd that pulsed and surged and jostled like a giant snaky organism. Within what seemed like minutes, maybe two thousand people were dancing and pressed into this amazing, spontaneous formation. Indeed, two actual funerals joined along the way, and it was quite intense: women went into ecstatic frenzies, men spasmed, children shouted "Yes!" and "Go On!"

Anyway, it was hot and exciting and hypnotic, totally captivating because the procession went on and on, winding through street after street. As an innocent New Yorker, I had somehow imagined that we'd be going around the block and back to the tent again, so I was somewhat surprised when the brass band walked on and on through the unfamiliar streets—a quarter mile, half a mile, three quarters of a mile.

After a good long mile, the musicians suddenly stopped, took off their headdresses, and announced, "Well, that's it, folks. This is where the money runs out." There was genuine rage in the crowd, women crying, men shouting. A mini-rumble and grumbling of outrage rippled through the assemblage.

The musicians had led us right up to a police barrier—wooden sawhorses and police cars blocked the street, and beefy officers stood with their arms folded.

Then, through all the chaos, there occurred a slow drifting of bodies, a traversing of the police line by nearly every white person in the crowd, as well as a very few people of color. And I realized that I knew nearly all those people who were drifting over behind the police barrier, because they were all fellow attendees at the very arts conference of which I too was a part, and they were beckoning to me, telling me to come over, cross over, to the other side.

Apparently the arts organization that had sponsored my trip to New Orleans had paid the $5,000 for the brass band permit. It had all been prearranged, to surprise us, to lead us like the pied piper from the spoken-word tent to the dinner afterward.

And, oh, the dinner. Beyond the police barrier was a narrow table that stretched for two long blocks, down a street of those beautiful old historic row houses for which the Eighth Ward is noted. It was a sit-down dinner for two hundred, one hundred people on one side of the table, one hundred on the other—so a very long, very dramatic table, set for a ten-course dinner, with candles and linens and crystal and waitstaff, set in the middle of this poor Black neighborhood, the residents sitting on their stoops as backdrop, like dark prophetic ghosts.

The dinner was billed as an art "happening," an "event," a "ritual feast" with "edible art," and had been crafted by a local entrepreneur. It was an amazing sight, the table shimmering in white light, extending onward as though to an infinity point—the end point of that infinity being another police barrier two blocks away, at the other end of the table. All around me arose a murmur of appreciative "oohs" and "ahhs" from the assembled artists and museum trustees and curators. The waiters scurried about furnishing the guests with local plum-glazed grilled alligator skewers "courtesy of Senator Sam Nunez" (who, rumor had it, had wrestled the beast to its death barehanded) and goblets of LaLeroux punch, described as a mixture of old New Orleans amber rum, brewed chicory, pressed ginger, fresh mint, local honey, and jalapeño. I got a copy of the menu before I left, and the names of the courses were intriguing. "At the Crossroads" consisted of absinthe in heart-shaped flowers, with vermouth, egg white froth, and hand-gathered, solstice-charged spring water. "Now Become Creole" consisted of Napoléon's roasted squab, heart of watermelon, and lucky black-eyed peas with 130 monk-made herbs, pickled rind compote, and popcorn sprouts. And the course labeled "Into Purity" consisted of chilled almond-milk soup with carbonated grape, and white chocolate–dipped sugarcane.

But, as I said, I did leave. I could not make myself sit down at that table. I couldn't quite work up an appetite beneath the weight, the simmering gaze of the people who actually lived there, gathered somberly on their stoops, little children on roller skates and bikes, gliding up and down the sidewalks, asking for samples from the caterers and being told that it was a private event on that public street, and that there wasn't enough. I left in a cloud of . . . something for which I have no name.

Having no idea where I was, I passed back to the other side of the police barrier and got on an empty bus, one of a fleet chartered to return guests to the hotel after the festivities. I convinced the driver to take me back early. I sat in the darkness, talking to the driver, who had been a driver the infamous night of the evacuation from the New Orleans Convention Center. She told me that the woman who stages these banquets—for there had been more than a few before this—was not really an artist, but a real estate agent, and that she was trying to bring artists into the Eighth Ward to rejuvenate it, gentrify it. And that those somber residents liken her events to Klan rallies. And that she for one—the bus driver, that is—did not like people who drank hand-gathered, solstice-charged spring water.

The bus driver told me stories about the night of the evacuation, that grievous diaspora to all points and nowhere, some destinations *still* unknown. She told me that the hardest moment was when she had to argue with a National Guardsman about letting a woman board the bus with her just-deceased, still-unwashed newborn. The National Guardsman kept calling the body a biohazard and refused to let her board unless she discarded the child, literally threw the body away. My bus driver said she'd convinced the Guardsman to let the woman wrap the child in the shroud of a plastic garbage bag and place the body in the baggage compartment under the bus.

She regaled me with even more such tales all the way back to my fancy hotel, where I tried to sleep amid the fluffy silken pillows, pondering this reiterated national narrative of forced migration, of homelessness and exile.

13

The Raw and the Half-Cooked

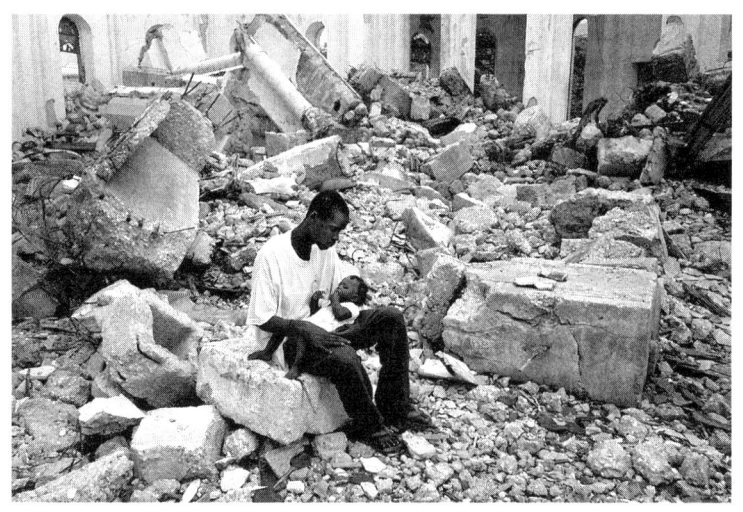

Fritz Robert Pierre-Saint, twenty-three, holds his daughter Christela Pierre-Saint among the ruins of the Cathedral of Our Lady of the Assumption, destroyed in the January 12, 2010, earthquake, in Port-au-Prince, Haiti

Photo by Dario Mitidieri/Getty Images

"How does one rewrite the chronicle of a death foretold and anticipated, as a collective biography of dead subjects, as a counter-history of the human, as the practice of freedom?" asks Saidiya Hartman in her lovely essay "Venus in Two Acts."

About three weeks after the 2010 earthquake in Haiti that killed an estimated 250,000 people, I met a woman in Boston's Logan Airport. She had just arrived from Port-au-Prince, and her story lingers in my mind. We were sitting on a bench waiting for a shuttle bus, and she wanted to talk. She really had to work at sparking that conversation, for I was deep in thought and not especially receptive. So it began slowly: she asked about the weather; I answered in monosyllables. She inquired about the timing of the shuttle's arrival; I gave her my copy of the schedule. She kept it going, however, offering small hints of engagement. She was on her way to stay with her son who lived in Rhode Island.

"Mmmm," I said.

She had three grandchildren.

"How nice."

Then she told me where she was coming from, and that she almost hadn't made it off the island amid all the chaos.

With that, she won my full attention. And when I followed her hints and asked the pertinent questions, she fell open, a river of sorrow, a rush of souls, an avalanche of death. So many dead, so many died, she said over and over. She had just gone outside to cook for the family, she had lit the fire in the *charbonnière*, the earth shifted, the buildings collapsed. She kept repeating the story; she had been sitting in her yard with the meat half-cooked, the earth shifted for an instant, the buildings collapsed. She told me the same story eight or nine times, each iteration with some new detail: she had seasoned the meat; the flowers were in bloom, her youngest daughter was doing her schoolwork. Then she looked over her shoulder, the earth moved, the house collapsed, and everybody died. All wiped out in the colossal rumbling of an instant.

Suddenly, the woman halted her terrible liturgy and the story took a turn out of nowhere. "You know what happened," she confided, lowering her voice. "The night before the earthquake there was a funeral for a nine-year old girl. In the middle of the service, she sat up in her coffin and said 'I'm too hot.' Then she jumped out, ran around the church three times and into the night."

With that, the woman fell silent. She did not speak another word until we parted.

"Here is a story," my grandmother used to begin her best tales, "that is and isn't true." And that's how I came to hear this woman's tale, this story straight from the book of the dead, or the day of the dead, or as my grandmother used to describe it, the night that has no eyes. Wombs and tombs tumbling open, the earth stalked by ghosts. For everything else she said that might have been accepted as factual, it was that supernatural image of the little girl rising from her coffin that brought home the horror and incalculable fear of the hellish night in Port-au-Prince—the bodies never found by families who remain nameless, the disorder that will bend and break an entire generation, the losses that will not be recorded, nor find their way to collective address, into the consciousness we call history—all the incomprehensible reversals of logic and illogic, the quick and the moribund, the active and the passive.

Once I began to hear her story as parable, it had a perfect coherence: It pointed to the enormity of that hole in time when the laws of man and nature had turned upside down, so that the dead became alive, and the alive became dead even as they were preparing to eat. That conjuration conveyed more vividly than all the political, media, and statistical accounts—combined—what we had encountered when we went out into the evening and we prepare the fire and the meat will be somewhere between raw and half-cooked and the world is suddenly suspended.

The closest I have come to that sort of suspension occurred when COVID hit the world. Now more than 15 million deaths later, I look back on those early days. The first COVID death in my cohort was a wonderful old friend who died on Monday, March 23, 2020. The shock hit me like a physical blow. The second death came less than a week later. There was no time to mourn. Then I became trapped in a season of funeral after funeral after funeral. Perhaps because I lived in New York City for so long and because New York City was the epicenter in those early days, hardly a day went by without some sort of bad news. I Zoom-sat with an old friend as she engaged in the cruelly named "live-stream viewing" of her mother's body. Then again for her father—she lost both within twenty-four hours. I sat a vigil for Lila Fenwick, the first African American woman to graduate from Harvard Law School, in 1956.[1] When I first started teaching at Columbia in 1991, I came as the first African American woman to join the faculty, and she just showed up in my office one day and introduced herself. She thought I might be lonely and very quietly stood by me, even auditing one of my classes, never saying very much; she was just there—giving me support and inspiration and nodding her approval. It was a much needed and very generous gift of . . . presence.

And of course that was what was hardest of all: the lack of human presence.

Philosopher Judith Butler writes of the "national melancholia" that proceeds from "disavowed mourning" for unremarked, "ungrievable deaths."[2] Indeed, I found the muffled isolation nearly intolerable. I worked remotely; I made myself Zoom with people every day. But screen presence is itself deadening. It's impossible to feel moods through Zoom; the passivity of the medium made me feel helpless. I hated teaching, talking, communicating through the mechanical mask that platforms offered, even as I knew I'd go mad (or more) without them. Home alone, I took Zumba online and yoga online, ordered food online, held friends' hands online, attended the philosophy department's weekly "happy hour" online (during which we morosely debated the existential meaning of happiness). I was scared to go much farther than once-weekly trips to the mailroom and the incinerator, during which I wore the equivalent of a burka (suddenly they seemed so sensible!) fashioned from plastic bags, and after which I took off all my clothes and gave thanks for having a washer and dryer in my apartment rather than having to use a shared laundry room. I tried to stay sane: I ordered an herb box to see if I could grow the color green. I bought a watercolor set to fight off boredom. I put (washable!) blue and pink streaks in my hair. I was so grateful to have a piano in my small space; as badly as I play, it was a particularly salutary release of anxiety. I tried to write every day, even though it was hard to focus. I talked to my therapist by Zoom. I went to a seder in Los Angeles by Zoom, to a Zoomed meditation circle in Montreal, and to mass with the pope, Zoomed from the emptiness in St. Peter's Square.

These were exceedingly strange times. I had a dream the night after the seder in which I was dressed like Big Bird, and I was the protagonist in a children's book titled *Chicken Little Misbehaves at the Seder*. I was flapping my wings and squawking: "I don't think the Red Sea is going to open up this time!" The last page of the book was Chicken-me standing on a roof holding a sign that said, Help! The water is rising!

My therapist says it didn't take much of her very great training to decipher this one. And then she very (*very*) patiently reminded me that, after all, this *was* the story of Passover. And although my brain seemed to have lodged faith narratives and material states of emergency in two very different halves of my consciousness, I found it comforting to try to rethink my fear in light of that. (I have a lot of trying left to do.)

These days, I spend time thinking about my own family's archive—and what of "mine" will find reception among others after I am gone. I think about the ethics of foregrounding and backgrounding the lives of friends and forebears whose effects have come into my possession less by will than by happenstance—neglect, untimely death, a mere forgetting to clean out the attic. I own these things now—diaries, letters, photos, scrapbooks, tickets, wish lists, bits of ribbon, pressed flowers. Some of these items are so intimate—I am never sure whether I am rescuing them from oblivion or whether I'm engaged in a gussied-up form of tomb raiding. Some friends have advised that I sell the archive: there is much interest in African America family histories. I decide to gather and donate the material instead.

Owning this trove of others' thoughts is like owning a body. It is a powerful thing, this ability to edit or make speak, to value or toss, to amputate whole episodes of a memory vault. What do the living owe the dead, and under what circumstances? What control ought the dead have over the living? What does integrity of the body really mean in the context of legal structures like wills and contracts and laws that incorporate business enterprises as a form of personhood?

What kind of respect do we owe each other in terms of reputational control, regulation of intimacy, and the veracities of memory versus the voracities of cost-benefit?

At now past seventy years of age, I am nervous about the future. I don't mean my own mortality, but the future of the world as I know it. I worry for the disappearing mollusks and crustaceans that used to be so plentiful in the waters where I grew up. I worry for the dwindling numbers of hummingbirds that visit my little red feeders. I worry for bees and bats and turkeys and deer. I worry about the dying trees—lindens and ash and maple and oak. I worry about the loss of what the lushness of spring used to smell like, the once-mossy taste of fresh water. It is not only that my senses have dulled with years; it's that mass extinctions are occurring so rapidly that those of us who are old enough—who are not really that old at all in geological time—can smell what is missing, can breathe and taste the encroaching losses of each little organism, each little wild thing, each little lively flavor that has gone missing, forever.

My grandfather was born in the 1880s to former slaves. He lived long and well into his nineties, probably because he was not one to sweat the small stuff. Spilled milk? "Who's going to remember in a hundred years?" he would snort. He said it often enough to make the contrarian in me determined to remember everything for at least a hundred years. And so I hung on to the stories he told about his own youth—times before cars, before plastics, before the Wright brothers, before the Panama Canal, even before Jim Crow laws. He died in the 1980s, having savored every second of life. He loved air travel, cameras, and Xerox machines. He rejoiced in the words of Martin Luther King.

My father was born in 1915, and despite five—count-'em, five—strokes remained still vibrant and funny till his death at ninety-nine. He was a technical editor back in the days of computer mainframes, back when Fortran and Cobol were the lingua franca of techno-nerds. Like my grandfather, he too shrugged off the little things with a curt "Who'll care in a hundred years?" He regaled my son with tales of automobiles that had to be cranked, of rumble seats and running boards. He recalled the regular lynchings when he was growing up. The integration of the army. The battle at Anzio. The etymology of the word *smog*.

Till the end, when it was very hard to find ink ribbons for it, my father typed letters on an old sticky-keyed Smith Corona typewriter. As I craft my own words on a brand-new Mac Pro, I am grateful for the strength that time and intergenerational engagement bring. I am a Black female law professor, something my grandfather could never have imagined in a hundred or a million years. And I am about to email these words to my editor through an invisible cushion of whooshing cyberspace, something my technical engineer father worked for but now won't see.

Across the table from where I sit, my son is worried about fossil fuels. It's not just gas or heating oil, he says anxiously. He ticks off things that are petroleum-based—from the telephone to his polyester windbreaker to the electrical plugs to the milk jug to his ballpoint pen. "How will humanity continue?" he asks with a glint of panic.

Like him I worry about the crossroads at which we stand, but I'm old enough to appreciate how quickly the course of events can change, for the worse to be sure, but also for the better, if only the will is there. A hundred years, I remind my son as I point him to the recycling bin with that empty Gatorade bottle he's hoisting toward the trash, is only a few decades younger than the combustion engine. If my father could remember the very first smog alert, then my son might live to see the haze subside and the heavens reemerge. Or so I pray. The human spirit is amazingly, unexpectedly resilient. One hopes the body may be as well.

My son and I chat, narratives and caesuras working together to create what is recognizable as hope. What is drawn forward in time or left unmentioned becomes winnowed into compelling koans, epigrams, memories, monuments, knowledge, epic, and myth. In its most formal sense, that winnowing is revealed as the source of our most creatively generative—as well as creatively destructive—rituals, ceremonies and holy repetitions. Stories and their ellipses become ceremonies of remembrance and forgetting, forgiveness of resentments, as well as fuel for revenge, instruction manuals for divisions premised on defenses of identity rooted in *not* being the other.

In his book *A Primer for Forgetting*, scholar and essayist Lewis Hyde recounts his own family's lineage.[3] Hyde observes that the "truth about who you are lies not at the root of the tree but rather out at the tips of the branches, the thousand tips."[4] He refers to a publication written by his grandmother in which she traces his forebears to one William Hyde, born in 1610, who came to the American colonies in 1633.

> Twelve generations separate me from William Hyde. I have two parents, four grandparents, eight great-grandparents. . . . My forebears in 1610 may number 2,048. Grandmother's book remembers William Hyde but forgets 2,047 other ancestors, including William's wife. To practice subversive genealogy means to forget the

idealism of a single forefather and remember these thousands. With that remembrance you must multiply the sense of who you are, multiply it until it disappears.[5]

Hyde thus recuperates the notion of disappearance as a form of healing, not merely as that which is suppressed from memory. He studies the circumstances that allow us to let go of memories because they are no longer important, as well as those circumstances so traumatic that whole societies rise up to sacralize the importance of "never forgetting." Disappearing in this sense is a devotional act of thinking things through to their end, a practice, perhaps like a form of Zen, that is central to a quiet soul, an untormented mind, and the ordinary pleasures of a happily uneventful life.

Michel Foucault observed that power

> doesn't only weigh on us as a force that says no, but that it traverses and produces things, it induces pleasure, forms knowledge, produces discourse. It needs to be considered as a productive network which runs through the whole social body, much more than as a negative instance whose function is repression.[6]

The most dangerous "production" of such circulation is the seductive slide between symbolic action—like speech, thought, writing—and actual actions like genocide. Indeed, the very etymology of "propaganda,"—Latin for "that which is to be propagated"—exhorts to hurried action; it is language or messaging that urges us to act. It convinces us that payback must be swift and deadly. Injustice is a practice.

In law, amnesty and statutes of limitation are two mechanisms devised to interrupt or quell bloodlust. Law professor Martha Minow observes that statutes of limitation are also a kind of forgetting, for amnesty is not merely forgiveness but forbearance.[7] And Hannah Arendt believed that "the power to forgive" provided a certain redemption from "the predicament of irreversibility": it requires not that we re-act, but rather that we act "anew and unexpectedly," creating a space "that allows people to step beyond themselves into something other than opposition."[8] To undo practices of injustice, therefore, requires un-practicing: a non-acting, or stopping for thought. It requires a hiatus in which the process we call "due process" may be done. In this context, "forgetting is a lack of action, not a lack of thought."[9] Our concept of legal amnesty, Lewis Hyde takes pains to point out, is rooted not in easy clichés about forgiving or forgetting, but in the hard work of severing "the otherwise reflexive link between thought and action."[10]

My grandmother always used to say, "Don't see too much." It was her advice for child-rearing as well as for grace in friendship, and it was the gentle equivalent of "Forget about it." It was her way of urging restraint, in not eternally sweating the small stuff. It was an injunction to give others space for creativity as well as folly, for forgiveness as well as error. Years later, I fear the expression might be heard as a kind of scolding mantra to "mind your own business," but my grandmother understood minding one's own business as a kind forgetting, as a species of tolerance, a willingness to turn one's attention to the things that matter. For her, as for Hyde, building community was about choosing to let go as well as finding purpose in coming together. It is a reciprocal process, the balance between honoring each other by never forgetting and honoring each other with amnesty. If remembering is a retention central in the meting out of justice, so also is the literal manumission of forgetting. As Hyde puts it, "To forget is to stop holding on, to open the hand of thought."[11]

It is a lovely turn of phrase, the opened hand of thought.

"There are two kinds of burials," Hyde writes. "In one, something is hidden because we can't stand to look at it; in the other, it is buried because we are done with it. It has been revealed and examined, and now it may be covered up or dropped for good. This latter is proper burial, burial after attention has been paid and funeral rites observed."[12] Hyde's framing inspires a voracious hunger for insight about how to repair a world in which desperation and death underwrite unprecedented levels of global diaspora. Assuming a proper burial, what is the function of the forgetting that follows no path but the present?

Getting old is sometimes like being a keeper of memories in which no one has any interest. It's like watching lives not just pass away but actively be erased. This was my feeling when I lost my father, a few weeks short of his hundredth birthday. I suppose this sensation of despair is a part of my mourning him.

My father was so devoutly well-mannered. In my last conversation with him, he was upset about the rudeness of the staff at the assisted living facility where he lived. The things he cited were relatively small things, about which they would have had no clue—like calling him by his first name and never saying please or thank you, or speaking to him in infantile singsong when he was physically weak but mentally sharp, or making him wear a sweatshirt because it's cheaper to launder than the suits and ties he preferred.

In the last year of her life, I visited my mother in the hospital, after she had suffered a fall. She cited how nice it was to have a call button by her bed, but that she would never ever use it. She waited agreeably for someone to come and get her out of bed, put her in her wheelchair, bring that magazine she couldn't reach. "They have so many people to attend to!" she said with sweet appreciation and much self-deprecation. She didn't want to impose. She asked no one for anything. "As your father said: I wake up in the morning. I'm breathing. The sun is shining. Amen." She said she was at peace, just cremate her when it's time: "It's modest, and eco-friendly."

But I was so unprepared to let either of my parents go. Their quiet unremarked exits just felt so wrong. It's like I made them up. They were in my head but nowhere else. My brain feels like an unattended reliquary. I can't sustain maintaining the memory of their lives all by myself.

My mother was nearly a hundred when she passed away, and very fragile. She had osteoporosis; movement was a perpetual risk. She was so deaf, I couldn't talk to her on the phone anymore. And her vision was so impaired, she had to use a huge magnifying glass to read. But her mind was all there, to the end. She was clever and funny and full of genteel wisecracks and ironic asides. Close to the end, I would watch her and my son sit with their arms around each other, laughing and recollecting. He had to shout in her ear; but the contact made her wonderfully chatty. She reminded him of tales about when he was little; my son would beam and say, "I remember, Grandma," and "You're my best friend, Grandma." She gave him and me ideas—not instructions, just suggestions, for that was my very polite mother—about what to do with her ashes and those of my father. There is a magical power in being in the presence of a beloved other. After my father died, my son and my mother and I all touched each other, with great awareness that this, too, might be for the last time. As the senses fade, the ability to feel another's presence, to just touch, seems like such a gift. Something is rendered from the body in such moments: a magical thing-in-the-room.

I grew up with people who told stories as though stories were symphonies. Everyone chimed in. Everyone had a voice, even the babies and even the demented—as long as you had any kind of remnant of a brain stem, you could hum along or clap. You sat and you listened, and when it was your time, you pitched in and harmonized with or around or contrapuntally. It's why I used to love singing in choruses, though I'm not much of a singer; and why I love Latin and African dance and Zumba, although I'm not much of a dancer. It's not about exercise: it's a form of joyous sensory collective expression, for which there seems very little opportunity these days. I suppose I'm very unfit for whatever world is now in the process of becoming. I like long storylines and narrative arcs that go back generations. I do not like a round-the-clock barrage of seven-second short thoughts, "disrupted" curricula, or 140-character cutoffs.

Anyway. I am looking out my window right now. It is a very high-priced and desirable long view. I see eighteen smokestacks, a densely packed rooftop garage of at least a hundred cars, an infinity of brick and steel and poured concrete; I see three building cranes, one improbably fat seagull resting on the wind, five airplanes lined up on a path toward the airport, and a little blue sliver of harbor peeking between a big, gray gas tank and what might be the back side of a convention center. I see a tiny bus moving from right to left at an impossible altitude—it must be on a high floor of a distant parking lot. I see a billboard of a tattooed hipster with the legend CAR PAYMENTS SUCK.

I can see no actual human beings from my window. My father, my mother, and all too soon me: this is the landscape into which we will all disappear.

I think of the German word *Waldeinsamkeit*. It refers to a feeling of being alone in a forest, a sense of becoming one with nature, with a force of life infinitely larger than oneself. This feeling of infinitude is not simply about the immediate sensory pleasure of wind, leaves, and birds; I think of it as a connection to time. It is a kind of awe, a sense of transport in looking into the bottomlessness of the Grand Canyon or up at a star-studded sky: an awareness of one's small size and brief life in planetary terms, a sensation of being cradled by a gentle yet indifferent vastness, an intricacy of layered creation whose holism speaks, resonates in our core so completely that we are effaced, stunned. One feels hidden from view yet merged seamlessly with one's surroundings. To be overcome in this sense means that we forget our words and ourselves as anything but odd molecules in the glorious stellations of immensity. This is a rare feeling in our noisy world of fame, mirrors, and 24/7 celebrity. It is the opposite of a selfie moment. It requires that we stand very still to listen and let go, resting with what Lewis Hyde terms the "perfectly useless." It's a stillness into which we allow ourselves to disappear.

14

Gathering the Ghosts

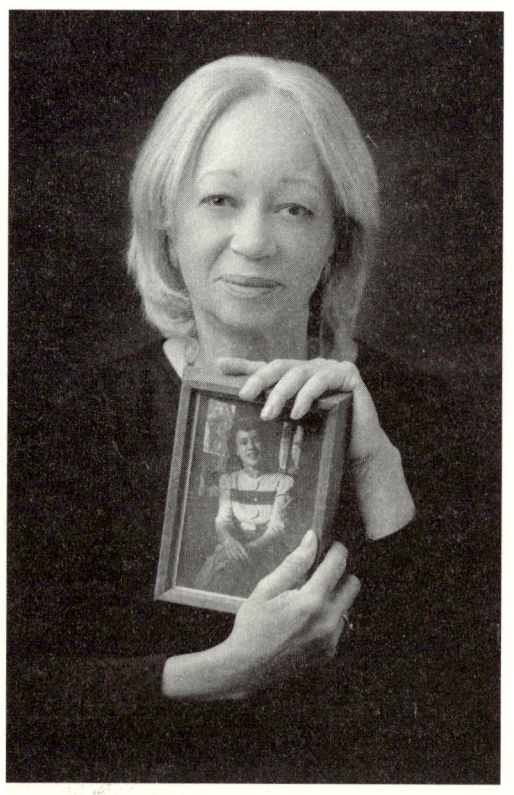

Jason M. Grow Photography

The Winter 2018 issue of *Radcliffe Magazine* featured a picture of me on its cover. Over the last few years, I've deposited more than a century's worth of photographs of my family into the Schlesinger Library, which is the women's history depository at Harvard University. I have photos of three of my great-grandparents, all born in slavery. I have missives from my uncle that describe life on the front during World War II. I have Boston Public School homework done by my aunts and uncles in the 1930s. I have my mother's diploma from Emerson College. I have newspaper clippings about an aunt who received her master's degree at the age of nineteen. And I have love letters from what was an unmentioned interracial marriage in the 1920s. It is rare for any American family, never mind an African American family, to have retained such a trove. I am lucky indeed.

The cover of that issue of the magazine depicted me cradling a photo of my late mother. Quite unexpectedly, this innocuous image brought me literally face-to-face with many of the ethical dilemmas at the center of a project archiving memories. It was surely very meaningful that my family's collection was so honored, but having my heavily made-up face dispersed to Radcliffe's far-flung readership brought with it a peculiarly personal sense of disembodiment. It was "me" but it was not "I." And the picture I was holding is of my late mother, when my mother was younger than I. Thus, this representation evoked for me the emotional layers at stake in the constitution of an archive, for there is a kind of quantitative magic in the ordering of things—in the imaginative assembly of images, in this gathering of ephemera that simultaneously quicken the dead and freeze-frame all life.

So there I was, on the cover, with pride of place all over campus. It was haunting to see this picture, of my mother in particular, out in the world, but also out of context. My hands around the frame of her face both presented her and protected her. It felt intimate and public—as though the photo were alive. There was a confusing promiscuity in seeing this me-object put to other ends: one dark and stormy evening, for example, I saw a homeless man in Harvard Square patching his cardboard tent with this cover. My glossily airbrushed face was subsumed into the paper's body, weight, texture, and durability. The substantiality of its high-grade bond put my life in context: the utility of my face as curtain, my persona a decorative detail. It seemed an oddly fitting encounter: the sense of disembodiment that haunted me throughout the explorations of this book had guided me to this final portal: the literal afterlife of papers.

It also forced me to think about some foundational difficulties involved in knowledge production and its preservation. Much of this archive was rescued from a dumpster into which it had been thrown by a team of earnest property managers hired to stage my parents' house—which had been in the family for over a hundred years—for sale. I fished it all out and put it in my apartment. This is my apartment after that fact:

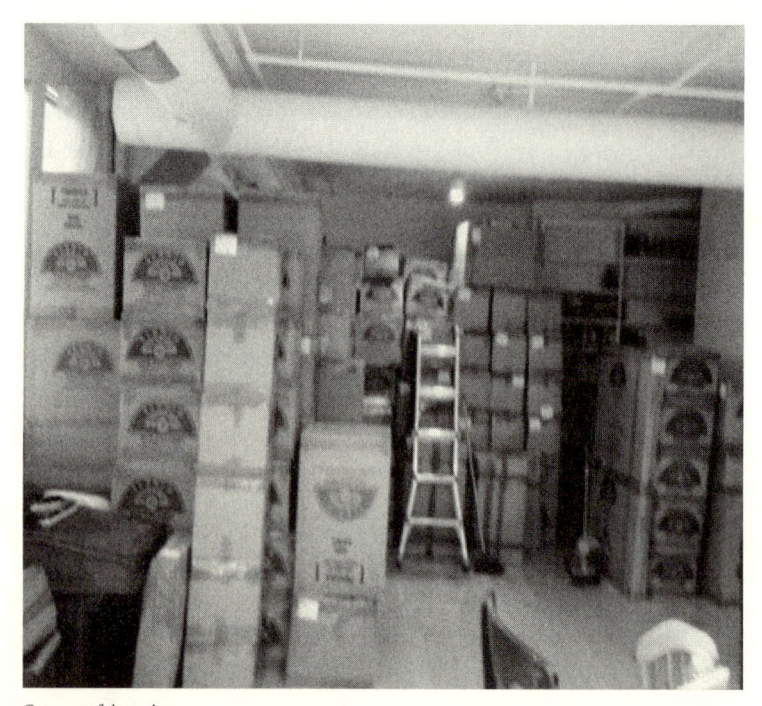

Courtesy of the author

Sorting through these boxes has called upon all my lawyerly talents of interpretative judgment and judicious discretion. At some much-too-obvious level, I suppose these materials could tell yet another tale of what W.E.B. Du Bois called the Talented Tenth. But their content also includes things that don't reference bourgeois accomplishment or assimilationist complacency alone. It includes stuff that was tossed into that attic for a reason.

So there are a number of dumpsters at work here. First, the literal, physical dumpster placed outside my parents' house and into which the anti-hoarding squad was tossing stuff from two floors up. Then there's the dumpster of self-censorship that some of this material represents—there is such secrecy and shame buried in it—secret yearnings, racial passing, infidelities. And then of course there's the dumpster of my own mind. There is great anxiety about what to release to Schlesinger, what beloved bodies to consign unto this "paper graveyard" (to borrow the title of scholar Eduardo Cadava's eloquent meditation on the accumulation of photographic art and its role in contemporary life[1]). What posthumous conundrums should I encrypt in the archival reliquary? What skins of existence should I allow others to paw through, to handle, out of my sight, at a time long after my death? I've had to really think about what not to give. What, if anything, to censor. The question that runs through my mind with each and every item is: How did it come to this, the maw of oblivion that is the dumpster?

For me the primal dumpster is slavery, the void into which so many lives disappeared without much trace. As I think about it, my ancestors' archive begins with the Emancipation Proclamation, with the outlawing of their bondage. It is at that moment that certain technologies became available to my great-great-grandparents. That's when anti-literacy laws were suspended, and it was no longer illegal for African Americans to learn to read and write. That's when photography was beginning to become available to amateurs. That's the point at which my foremothers and -fathers spilled out of the places and plantations that had bred and contained them, that's when they lied, charmed, walked slowly or ran fast, or otherwise got themselves out of the Deep South, first a few and then in a rush, headed northward to Boston, center of abolitionism, however they could. They became first-class tricksters to liberate themselves, and they picked up pens, paper, and typewriters and began to document the ineffability of themselves with a full-blown vengeance of expressive self-inscription.

The word *archive* comes from the Greek *arkheion*, meaning the house of a public administrator, a center of governance, lists, records, and rule making. I'm a lawyer, after all, so there is a part of me that does think of an archive in that rather positivistic and orderly way: a repository of transparent "evidence" from which "what happened" may be reconstructed with enough tape and tweezers and a big enough magnifying glass. Am I not the proverbial "handmaiden to history"? Isn't it my role merely to dust off the documents and arrange them prettily, like specimens under glass?

Many philosophers—Avery Gordon, Saidiya Hartman, Jacques Derrida—have written about the social life of archives, the busy-ness and noisiness of artifacts. And because that social life is filled with karmic irony, I was literally in the archive room of Schlesinger Library when I received word that my mother had passed away, on October 3, 2017. Suddenly, I was living the afterlife in a quite overpoweringly mystical way. These papers became a gathering, a familiarity, a nest of faces, a syntactical family, a tattered, much-handled sensorium, a ghostly mirror.

And there were voices. Bereavement does that, I suppose. All sorts of voices bloomed within me, but also beyond me, like a gentle aura. It was like looking at a jigsaw puzzle I thought I'd assembled, but suddenly there were thousands of extra pieces, and it became an assemblage with no borders and an endless number of combinations. It was a bit of a Hansel and Gretel experience, those voices: *Here is a trail of breadcrumbs*, they said. *This is the way to find us. This will lead you back in time. This will lead you forward. We are just behind this tree. We will be waiting in the clearing. You may see us in the morning. Look for a lesson hidden in the cupboard. And: there's an unbreakable law you will want to know about, lurking just beneath the bed.*

I have always thought of reality as a present tense. But in the archive, reality has leached all over the geography of time. In my mind, time begins with emancipation from slavery. But that temporal arc coexists alongside the reign of Great-Aunt Mary; as well as side by side with the dominion of the Cambridge cousins, which overlaps with my father's extended rule, as well as the still-reverberating echo of my mother's voice. Each of these timelines is a completely different world.

All of this leaves me feeling porous, unsettled, having lost the coherence of an identity I had thought of as my own. It brings felt meaning to the koan that novelist and Zen master Ruth Ozeki frequently cites as her meditative inspiration: "What did your face look like before your parents were born?"

I have spent a good deal of time recently thinking about how archives intersect with knowledge production. What does all this paper do—this stuff I keep shoveling into the bowels of the Schlesinger? We live, we die, and so it goes. From dust to being the soggy patchwork in a homeless stranger's tent and then back to dust. This is a question of representation, I suppose: what part of a life after life lives on as "papers"? What fiction will emerge, what wormholes to the future? Saidiya Hartman calls the method of the archive "critical fabulation" and has observed that "the question—who are you?—is indistinguishable from one's status as a social problem."

If *Radcliffe Magazine* made me lovely, this is what I looked like to the *Daily Mail* in 1996, which denounced me as a "single Black mother" of "slave stock":

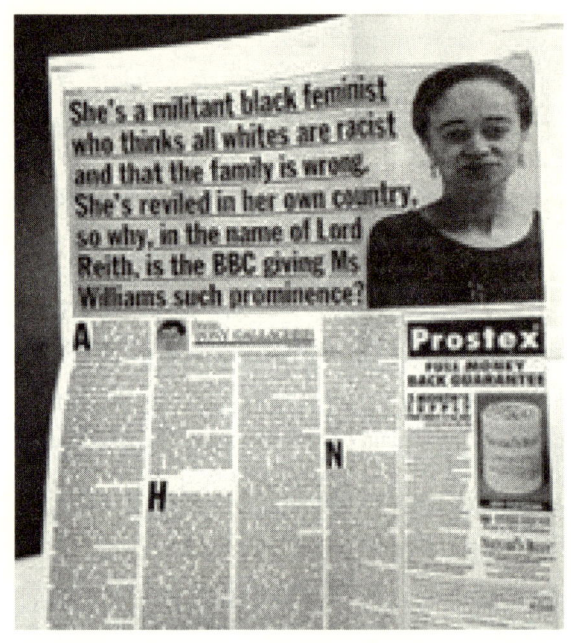

Courtesy of the author

(Note the way they positioned my portrait atop a bottle of Prostex, a health supplement for prostate problems. "Full money back guarantee.")

Seriously, this was a painful representation. I considered leaving it out of the Schlesinger repository. Kind of the equivalent of what my Great-Aunt Mary did to some of her less-flattering photos: she used to deploy a pair of cuticle scissors and very carefully pare her image out of the picture, leaving a blank white square where her head once was.

I've decided not to do that, at least as a rule, for this is how history gets put into the dumpster. Ultimately the very suppression leaves a void that will surely haunt us. Jacques Derrida's extraordinary essay "Archive Fever," exhorts us to remember the future.

Nonetheless, we're all implicated in withholding as oblivion. Indeed, it is precisely those small acts of calculated forgetting that make archiving a matter of social history. To record-keep or not to record-keep is a ritual of information management—of remittance or rejection, of the politics of the gatekeepers. In other words, there are choices to be made, even by me. Do I kill some stories? Amputate a few bits so no one will notice?

Somewhere in the boxes, there's a trove of love letters from my father to a woman not my mother. I have no idea why he kept them. They are quite beautifully written, so I suppose it might have been his considerable vanity. I am struggling to figure out if vanity and infidelity should be included—whether it betrays the memory of my father, or if it makes him more complexly human; whether it feeds a stereotype of rapaciousness, or if it invades the privacy he sought in life.

It is hard to navigate these challenges of representational ethics. And it's obviously not just about letters and photos, but about all the complex kinds of pictures that emerge from the entanglement of images and voice, correspondence and culture, temperament and time.

Some years ago, I lost the audition to record the Audible.com version of my memoir *Open House*.[2] The description on the packaging for the CD of *Open House* says: "[Patricia Williams's] voice is powerful, provocative, and utterly charming." But in fact it's not my actual voice. A very talented professional actress won the role of speaking me. She did a fine job, and her delivery was probably much better than I could have done—although I had to learn to hear myself in her, to own this rendering of my words. I was told that the reason I failed the audition was that my voice "did not sound Black enough."

The voice that is not always heard as mine resounds beyond me, both digital and disconnected. I think of Echo, the nymph who always had to have the last word, and who was cursed unto death by the inexpressible and repetitious, her last words mouthed by others.

Two of the most precious images I've found in the dumpster trove are photos of relatives who were born slaves. This is Peter Williams, my paternal great-grandfather, in what must have been his late nineties—he lived to be over a hundred.

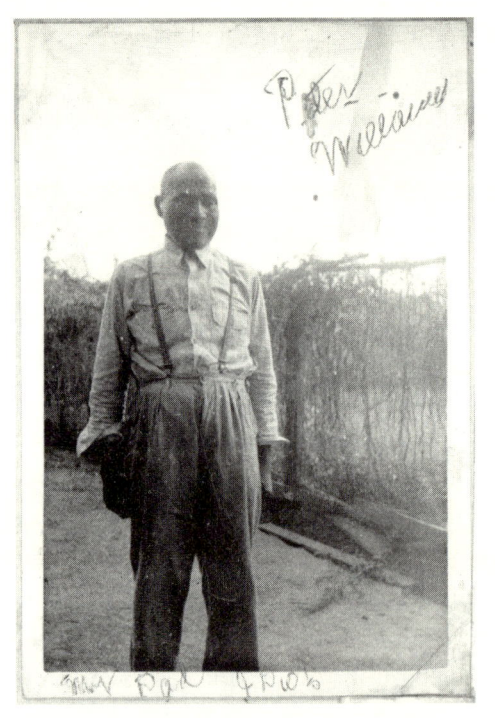

Schlesinger Library, Radcliffe Institute, Harvard University

He was born in slavery, and was in his seventies when he walked away from the plantation, so slowly that no one noticed. We call him the walkaway slave, and my son is named after him. He had a superpower that many Black men today are having to learn to harness, for better or worse: that of being present in the world, while steeling oneself into slow unnoticeability. No sudden moves, just blending on in while walking really, really quietly down that road. (This is perhaps "passing" of a different sort than we sometimes think.)

Anyway. Old Peter walked to freedom and started a lumber mill. Freedom suited him well. He got married in his late seventies, learned to read in his eighties, had a family of eight children, the eldest of whom was my paternal grandfather. On the next page is a photo of my paternal great-grandmother, Old Peter's wife. I do not know her name.

I also have a very fragile photo of my maternal great-grandmother,

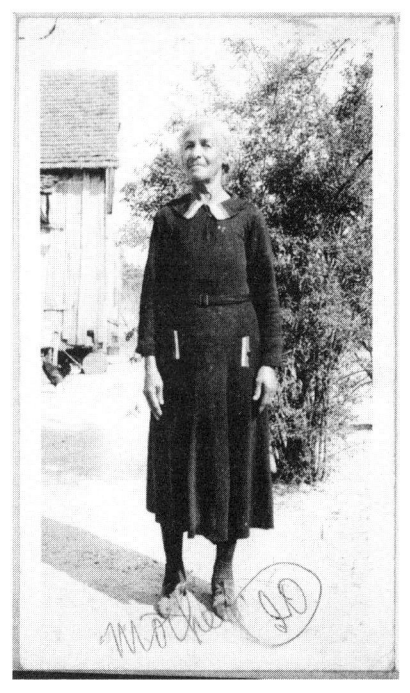

Schlesinger Library, Radcliffe Institute, Harvard University

Mattie Rose Miller, also born into slavery. She was taken from her mother to be raised as a "house slave." She was still a child when Emancipation set her free. I would guess the photo was taken in the 1890s or around the turn of the century, when she might have been in her thirties or forties. It is a professional portrait, taken in a studio, and she appears grave but prosperous, dressed in a fashionably embroidered dress with a high-necked lace collar, topped off with a large late-Victorian or Edwardian hat. She is carrying a version of the then-popular hybrid parasol/umbrella known as an *en tout cas*.

Mattie Rose's mother was a slave named Sophie; and Sophie is the subject and the starting place of my book *The Alchemy of Race and Rights*.[3] Sophie was twelve when she gave birth to Mattie Rose. Mattie Rose's father was white, a lawyer and a judge named Austin Miller, who legally "owned" Sophie, and whom my family remembers as "the master" rather than as kin. Austin Miller was in his thirties when he purchased Sophie from somewhere in Kentucky. She was eleven years old at the time of that purchase, and he wasted no time at all in breeding her.

I know a lot about Austin Miller because his papers—his property holdings, his judicial accomplishments, the names of his white wife and white children—his "legitimate" family—are preserved in the National Archives in Washington, DC.

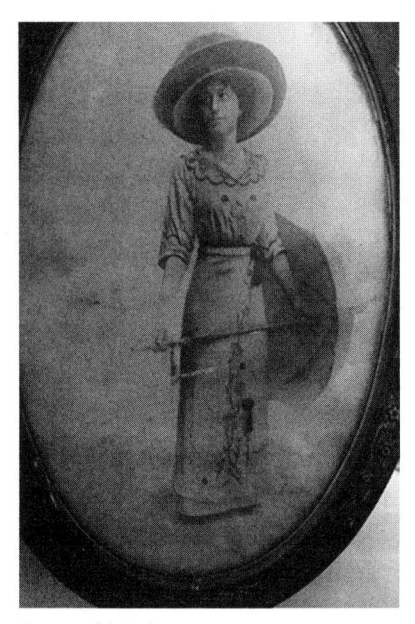

Courtesy of the author

By all such accounts, he was a wealthy and respected man.

I know very little about the child who was my great-great-grandmother Sophie. I mourn not having pictures of her. I mourn her. I am committed to rendering her into existence, to make a mark on her behalf, to give her form and face, to cherish her in the not-national archive of my memory. And so I dream her, but she is unthinkable. In his book *Silencing the Past*, Michel-Rolph Trouillot writes, "The unthinkable is that which one cannot conceive within the range of possible alternatives, that which perverts all answers because it defies the terms under which the questions were phrased." But there's a placeholder for Sophie in my mind. I know that imagining my great-great-grandmother's face, while irresistible, is really much too easy, and overly sentimental. She is, indeed, the face my face looked like before my parents were born.

I once heard the filmmaker and theorist Trinh T. Minh-ha speak about how she approaches her projects: "We have to walk not only with those whom we can see. We need to learn to walk with those who have disappeared."

Meanwhile Sophie's daughter, my maternal great-grandmother Mattie Rose, married a man named William Ross, who was not born in slavery, but had been raised somewhere in Canada, we think in Quebec. He was a very fine musician who played with some sort of band that had traveled to Memphis to play, and that's how he met my great-grandmother. They had seven children, including my grandmother, born in 1884. Their two sons—my great-uncles Richard and Rufus—were also musicians, spending their careers playing with W. C. Handy's blues band.

I am fortunate enough to have grown up with lots of stories passed down about these great-grandparents, but I had never seen their faces before combing through my trove of boxes. The sudden apparition of their oddly familiar features has been so startling, so jolting, so magical that I sometimes feel as though I am hallucinating. It is as though their images had coiled upward from the scrapbook, like smoke, and entered my body.

Their presence has bloomed within me, but also beyond me, like a gentle aura. There is something dark and inexplicable yet entirely illuminating in the eeriness of this encounter with ghosts. I try to read their lives from fragments, the tea leaves of their long-gone presence. I

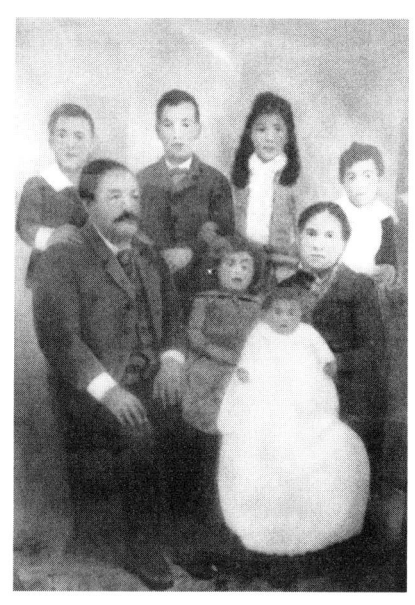

Courtesy of the author

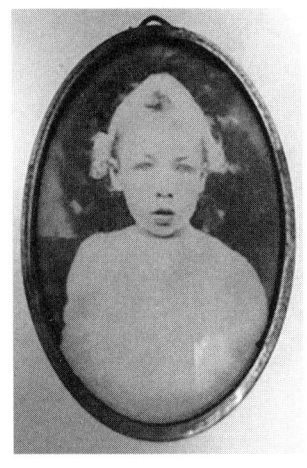

Courtesy of the author

listen to W. C. Handy's "Saint Louis Blues" and listen for the piano, the violin, the guitar—these were the instruments my great-uncles played. I look at old photos from albums and newsreels and try to pick them out.

Still, in my combing through the photos, much has been lost. In the days before my mother's death, I was sending her questions, not all of which she got around to answering. The archive is filled with questions and unidentified faces. For example, I have a faded image of my Uncle Carl as a very young child, in an oval frame, taken sometime in the early 1900s. My late cousin Marguerite told me who it was. I look at this picture and realize no one on earth will remember who this is—I am quite literally the only one who still knows. The image is very tenuously bound to me and me alone in the universe.

I suppose this ache for recuperative connection across generations, for the echo of no-longer-present bodies in living ones, is ritualized by such cultural phenomena as the Day of the Dead, when spirits rise from the grave to join their living loved ones for food and drink. If those spirits are forgotten by the living, if the stories of them cease to be told in the real world, then they disappear. When no human is left who will preserve your memory, or make a shrine of your pictures, or lay out the food that symbolizes communion with the living—then that's when you do actually pass away, forever.

I spend a lot of time thinking about photos without captions, without stories, without narrative or history. I fear that images alone risk becoming strangers, profiles, free-floating signifiers, landscapes upon which viewers inevitably project whatever they think they see.

Whether that is an essentially good thing or a bad thing is a freighted question for me. Can a picture stand on its own? Must it?

Theorist Fred Moten asks: What is "the sound that precedes the image?" Indeed. How does one write shading and background, soundscape and understanding, into and around each image?

In this photo, from 1942, my paternal grandfather and Aunt Margaret and Uncle Lonnie and a family friend are all standing in a row eating slices of watermelon. I become anxious about its display: it *needs* me to interpret it. I live with the fear that if it is just seen by the public at large, they'll tend to see a random line of Black people with large slices of watermelon, smiling—"grinning," they might even say—while they consume a highly overdetermined fruit, shamelessly!

But I knew these people, I know the backstory, I grew up hearing their voices: this is a picture of four doctors poking fun at the stereotype. Note that my grandfather is wearing a full three-piece suit in the picture. He holds his slice with dignity, with the tips of his fingers, the graceful hands of the surgeon he was. If you look closely, they are all quite well-dressed, all elegant professionals—four Black doctors asserting that hard-earned status with insistent and relentless pride, never letting anyone forget the dignity of that title, Doctor—mocking the mockery of *The Birth of a Nation* and blackface Disney cartoons.

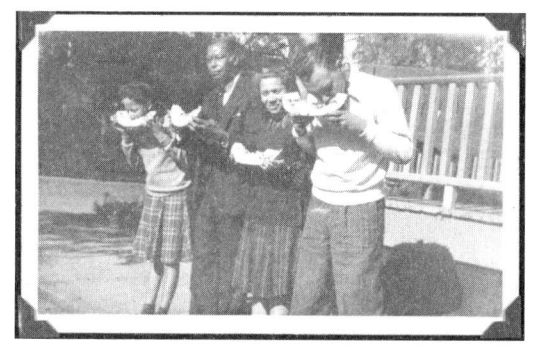

Schlesinger Library, Radcliffe Institute, Harvard University

Among family, this photo was something to laugh about, but in the archive it may have to stand alone.

I hand over these pictures of the past as a gift to the future. But so much needs translation, just as this photo needs context to read it as a facetious statement about how to enjoy life, how to subvert the constraints of respectability and amuse oneself with the forbidden genus *Citrullus lanatus*, the fruit of disreputability, while pantomiming the irredeemable practices of leisure, lounging, laziness, and lust. So, providing not merely identification, but the sound and circumstance for these photos has felt pressing to me.

Pattern recognition, of bodies and part of bodies, is another game of the archive: there is much repetition of poses and themes and family resemblances. This is a photo of my paternal Aunt Margaret, circa 1922, with her dolls:

Somewhere, lost to time and the clutter of my storage unit, is a photo of me, around the age of three, with my dolls, The tilt of my head, my squinting into the sun—is an eerie echo of Aunt Margaret's pose decades before. Even our dolls are identical. I look at our child-selves and see in these images a long intergenerational history of little Black girls playing with exclusively white dolls. But I also look at us and see that I wear my aunt's face. It is as though we are time-traveling twins.

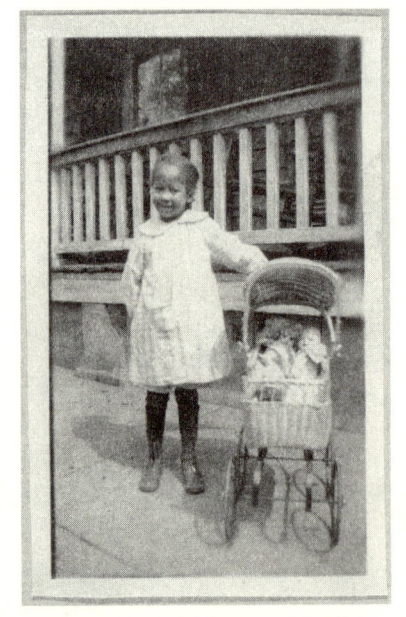

Schlesinger Library, Radcliffe Institute, Harvard University

By the same magic token, my mother in the moments after her

death became an entirely different person. She, the mother I knew, was gone. Instead my mother in death wore the face of my grandmother and great-grandmother, as though they had swooped in and were occupying her body. They looked at me through her, appraising across time and generation. The philosopher Emmanuel Levinas wrote that it is the face-to-face encounter that inspires one to give to and serve others, for it "involves a calling into question of oneself, a critical attitude which is itself produced in the face of the other."

My mother was a magnificent storyteller. When I was growing up, her stories always sat outside our bodies, a magical thing-in-the-room, protecting us from goblins, reassuring us, making us laugh. It's as though we could pick them up and put them on, and they'd live forever as long as we wore them. They shimmered. Those shared stories composed us, rooted us, made us consistent and satisfied.

In this sense, the complicated visual effigies in the archive have taken up residence within me like marvelous secret agents of love, sadness, healing, and heroism. Their shapes have insinuated themselves as armatures for carrying on, brave imaginaries for the mind and heart. They have become ethical reference points in the seeping disfigurements of trauma, rage, cruelty, and death. They speak figuratively. The echo of their voices is an epiphany of repair, assurance to lost children of their place in worlds to come.

In Ōtsuchi, Japan, there is something called the telephone of the wind. In 2010, a seventy-two-year-old man named Itaru Sasaki lost his cousin. To comfort himself, he set up a phone box high on a hill overlooking the water. There's a rotary phone inside that is "connected to nowhere." Because there is no wire, Sasaki speaks of the wind carrying his voice, from the living to the dead. Tens of thousands have come to commune with the dead by wind phone—this surreal link between the grieving and the lost, this commitment to connection when connection has been cut.

Surrealism is a movement designed to make art of such fugue states, a search to make meaning of the irrational, the inexpressible. Just so, the archive is surreal. It is inhabited by objects that speak, silence that writes volumes, and the life of witness-without-words. As I put things in, I do so in the name of releasing these intimate bodily renderings into an uncertain future, a zeitgeist. A time-spirit far beyond me. I do yearn to control them. Sometimes I flatter myself with the privilege of inscription: *The dead are mine. I write them in and out of being. I talk over them, behind them, through them. And they speak to me. They speak through me.* Even as they are perfectly indifferent to me.

Such is the conceit of archiving as a social process. I yearn to have future beings see me and my wonderful forefathers and -mothers. *We were all here!* I wish them to live in social imagination more fully than many of them were able to while on the planet. And so I need to explain. I am constantly explaining. I am always looking for the right words, the right accent, the perfect analogy, the smoothest homology, the felt connection, the link that sparks a mental orgasm of humanizing recognition. I throw myself at this task over and over again. It's Promethean. It's obsessive, compulsive, disordering. But I also like to think of it as principled folly, moral insistence, an endeavor of reassembly and healing remembrance for the long haul.

Acknowledgments

This book has evolved over a long and uneven arc of time, spanning the traumatic division between pre- and post-pandemic lockdown years. I am deeply indebted to Gail Hochman, my longtime agent, and to the many friends, colleagues, and institutions who supported me through the fragmentation of that era. At the top of that list are the remarkable Diane Wachtell, founding editor of The New Press, whose enthusiasm for and faith in this project allowed it to materialize; and Rachel Vega-DeCesario, whose infinitely patient editorial labor hammered it (and me) into shape. Other New Press staff I would like to thank are Emily Albarillo, Maury Botton, Fran Forte, and Nia Abram. I am also grateful for Karol Kepchar at Akin Gump, whose guidance on the artwork proved invaluable.

I was also graced by the support of my singularly talented former research assistant Julia Mendoza, whose tireless flow of great feedback, great ideas, and great good humor kept me going, year after very long year; my kind and generous teaching assistant, Ana Souffrant; my spectacular editors at *The Nation Magazine* including Katrina vanden Heuvel, Don Guttenplan, Atossa Araxia Abrahamian, and Shuja Haider; my insightful friend and editor at the *A-Line Journal*, Richard Blint; Hamilton Fish, wise publisher of *The Washington Spectator*; the brilliant team of scholars associated with the *Logische Phantasie Lab*, especially co-directors Daniela Gandorfer, Zulaikah Ayub, and Tanja Traxler.

I am grateful to my former colleagues at Columbia University by whom I have been long inspired, particularly Elizabeth Emens, Marianne Hirsch, Robert Pollack, Amy Pollack, Marcia Sells, and Kendall Thomas; my current colleagues at Northeastern University who have made teaching there a delight, including Margaret Burnham, James Hackney, Adam Hosein, Jonathan Kahn, Lori Lefkowitz, Angel Nieves, and Wendy Parmet. I am especially indebted to my diverse friends and mentors in the arts who have taught me much about media, visual culture, graphic design, and aesthetics: Josh Begley, David Birkin, Eduardo Cadava, Mel Chin, Teju Cole, Peter Goodrich, Max Houghton, Bouchra Khalili, Bradley McCallum, Linda Mills, Nicholas Mirzoeff, Anna Deavere Smith, and Autumn Womack. I thank my various "writing buddies" with whom the discipline of regular meetups has kept me focused: Moya Bailey, Kristin Bumiller, Patricia Ewick, Alice Hearst, Eunsong Kim, Martha Minow, Susan Silbey, and Martha Umphrey. Similar appreciation must go to my special "walking while talking" friends, with whom invaluable thought-connections have been made during conversations that began as small wandering tugs of curiosity, then progressed to sudden streaks of golden illumination: Jessie Allen, Richard R. W. Brooks, Troy Duster, Cynthia Dwork, Michele Goodwin, Sandra Grymes, Evelynn Hammonds, Anita Hill, the late, great Sheldon Krimsky, Caroline Light, Jane Lipson, Osagie Obasagie, Constance St. Louis, and Ann Stoler.

Lastly, I could not have finished this book without the support of the following entities and institutions: the Andy Warhol Foundation, the Colloquium in Legal, Political and Social Philosophy at New York University, the Institute for Arts and Civic Dialogue at New York University, the Institute for Critical Social Inquiry at The New School, the Nation Institute, the Northeastern University Humanities Institute, the Princeton Atelier, the Radcliffe Institute for Advanced Study, and the University of Richmond School of Law Faculty Colloquium.

Notes

1. Detachment

1. School of Castile and León, *Saints Cosmas and Damian Healing a Christian with the Leg of a Dead Moor*, 1460–1480, private collection.
2. Frederick Douglass, *The Narrative of the Life of Frederick Douglass, An American Slave: Written by Himself*, published at the Anti-Slavery Office, No. 25 Cornhill, Boston, 1845.
3. Jean-Luc Nancy, "The Intruder," in *Corpus* (New York: Fordham University Press, 2008).
4. Nancy, "Intruder."
5. *Finders Keepers*, Firefly Theater & Films, 2015.
6. Wood's sense of attachment is in line with a long history of body parts revered as sacred relics. See: Jamie Kreiner, *The Wandering Mind: What Medieval Monks Tell Us About Distraction* (New York: Liveright, 2023), recounting the story of St. Simeon, who purportedly cut off his own infected foot in order to be less distracted while praying, and was said to have reassured his severed limb that they would be reunited in the afterlife.
7. Melena Ryzik, "'Finders Keepers,' the Story of a Gnarled Leg and the Lives It Altered," *New York Times*, September 18, 2015.
8. "Judge Mathis Show Scene Movieclips," https://www.youtube.com/watch?v=XPhVzIgYjhc.
9. The Declaration of Independence, 1776, National Archives of the United States of America.
10. *Dred Scott v. Sandford*, 60 U. S. 393 (1857).
11. Matthew Salafia, "Searching for Slavery: Fugitive Slaves in the Ohio Valley Borderland, 1830–1860," *Ohio Valley History* 8, no.4 (Winter, 2008). See also: Levi Coffin, *Reminiscences of Levi Coffin, the Reputed President of the Underground Railroad* (Cincinnati, 1876; New York: Arno Press, 1968).

12. P. S. Bassett, "A Visit to the Slave Mother Who Killed Her Child," *American Baptist*, Fairmont Theological Seminary, Cincinnati, Ohio, February 12, 1856.

13. Bassett, "Visit to the Slave Mother."

14. Jordan Belfort, *The Wolf of Wall Street* (New York: Bantam Press, 2008), 104.

15. "The Story Behind DeSantis's Migrant Flights to Martha's Vineyard," *New York Times*, October 4, 2022, l.

16. Stephanie Lai, "Buses of Migrants Arrive at Kamala Harris's Home on Chrismas Eve," *New York Times*, December 25, 2022.

17. "Saints Cosmas and Damian," *Encyclopædia Britannica*, 1988.

18. Nebojša J. Jovic and Marios Theologou, "The Miracle of the Black Leg: Eastern Neglect of Western Addition to the Hagiography of Saints Cosmas and Damian," *Acta medico-historica adriatica* 13, no. 2 (2015): 329–44, abstract available at PubMed, pubmed.ncbi.nlm.nih.gov/27604202.

19. Literary theorist Leah Whittington explores the way history comes to us in pieces, perpetually unfinished, always in fragmentary form. Her ongoing project "Antiquity Made Whole: Completions and Renaissance Literary Culture" focuses on practices of "adding to, carrying forward or finishing" ancient texts that have survived—but only partially—and "the role of damaged or fragmentary works in spurring new artistic creations." See, Leah Whittington, "The Mutilated Text," in *The Unfinished Book*, ed. Deidre Lynch and Alexandra Gillespie (Oxford: Oxford University Press, 2020), 429–443.

20. Jared Bland, "It's 'Scary' Watching Aspects of Her Fiction Come to Life, Says Margaret Atwood," *Toronto Globe and Mail*, August 24, 2013.

2. Amputation

1. Richard Sandomir, "Williams Children Agree to Keep Their Father Frozen," *New York Times*, December 21, 2002.

2. "Ted Williams Frozen in Two Pieces," *CBS News*, December 20, 2002.

3. Brian Michael Murphy, *We the Dead: Preserving Data at the End of the World* (Chapel Hill: University of North Carolina Press, 2022).

4. "The Truth About 'Medbeds'—a Miracle Cure That Doesn't Exist," *BBC News*, December 26, 2022.

5. "The Truth About 'Medbeds.'"

6. Christine Hauser, "Judge Cites 1849 Slavery Law in Ruling Embryos Can Be Considered Property," *New York Times*, March 16, 2023.

7. Opinion Letter, *Honeyhline Heidemann v. Jason Heidemann*, CL-2021-0015372, Nineteenth Judicial Circuit of Virginia, February 8, 2023.

8. Opinion Letter, *Heidemann*.

9. Clifford Ward, "Judge Dismisses Lawsuit over Downers Grove Sperm Bank Mistake," *Chicago Tribune*, July 21, 2016l.

10. Ward, "Downers Grove Sperm Bank Mistake."

11. "Jennifer Cramblett: I Can't Let Them Do This to Another Family," *NBC News*, October 1, 2014.

12. "Cramblett: I Can't Let Them." See also: Nicole Chung, "The Family Who Tried to End Racism Through Adoption," *The Atlantic*, April 2023.

13. "The Daily Show Extended Interview with Bill O'Reilly," YouTube, Comedy Central, October 16, 2014.

14. Cheryl Harris, "Whiteness as Property," *Harvard Law Review* 106, no. 8 (June 1993): 1707–91.

15. Rachelle Blidner, "Legacy of Exclusion Is Tough to Shed," *Newsday*, November 17, 2019.

16. Joshua Ruff, "Levittown: The Archetype for Suburban Development," *American History Magazine*, December 2007. See also: David Kushner and Tavia Gilbert, *Levittown: Two Families, One Tycoon, and the Fight for Civil Rights in America's Legendary Suburb* (Walker Books, 2009).

17. Kushner and Gilbert, *Levittown*.

18. *Shelley v. Kraemer*, 334 US 1 (1948).

19. Bruce Lambert, "Study Calls L.I. Most Segregated Suburb," *New York Times*, July 5, 2002.

20. "Levittown, New York," World Population Review, 2023. See also: "Levittown CDP, New York," United States Census Bureau, 2022.

21. Camille Gear Rich, "Contracting Our Way to Inequality: Race, Reproductive Freedom, and the Quest for the Perfect Child," *Minnesota Law Review* 104 (2020): 2375–2469.

22. Cover, *New York Post*, March 22, 2007.

23. Todd Venezia, "Black Baby Is Born to White Pair," *New York Post*, March 22, 2007, p. 6.

24. Venezia, "Black Baby."

25. J. Martinez, "What a Mess, Baby," *New York Daily News*, March 22, 2007.

26. Matthew Guterl, *Skinfolk: A Memoir* (New York: Liveright, 2023). See also: Nicole Chung, "The Family Who Tried to End Racism Through Adoption," *The Atlantic*, April 2023.

27. Guterl, *Skinfolk*; and Chung, "The Family Who Tried."

28. Guterl, *Skinfolk*; and Chung, "The Family Who Tried."

3. Lone Ranger

1. McGinnis, "'Prince' Leonard."
2. McGinnis, "'Prince' Leonard."
3. Fugitive Slave Act of 1850, Library of Congress.
4. Individual Freedom Act, more commonly called the Stop the Wrongs to Our Kids and Employees [WOKE] Act, Florida House Bill 7, 2022.
5. "An Act Relating to Abortion, Including Abortions After Detection of an Unborn Child's Heartbeat; Authorizing a Private Civil Right of Action," Texas House Bill 8, 2021.
6. "An Act Relating to Abortion."
7. Jordan Liles, "False Rumor Claims Paul Pelosi Brought Attacker Home from Gay Bar," Snopes, October 31, 2022.
8. Kate Conger, Davey Alba, and Mike Baker, "False Rumors That Activists Set Fires Exasperate Officials," *New York Times*, September 10, 2020.
9. Gavin Butler, "Teen Who Sold a Kidney for an iPhone Is Now Bedridden for Life," *Vice*, January 28, 2019.
10. Butler, "Teen Who Sold a Kidney."
11. Patricia J. Williams, "Babies, Bodies, and Buyers," *Columbia Journal of Gender and Law* 33, no. 1 (2016): 11–24.
12. Seeking, https://www.seeking.com.
13. Miriam Wasser, "Sugar Daddies Pay Tuition for Hundreds of ASU Students," *Phoenix New Times*, January 14, 2016.
14. "ASU Students Explain Why They Want Sugar Daddies," *Phoenix New Times*, September 11, 2013.
15. "Dr. Phil: Sugar Baby Students," https://www.youtube.com/watch?v=MnIuEOeZXUc.
16. Tyler McCall, "Sara Ziff Has Spent the Last Decade Changing the Fashion Industry—and She's Just Getting Started," *Fashionista*, February 14, 2022.

17. Laia Garcia-Furtado, "Model Alliance Founder Sara Ziff Accuses Former Miramax Head of Rape," *Vogue*, April 7, 2023.

18. Abha Bhattarai, Dan Keating, and Stephanie Hays, "What Does It Cost to Raise a Child?" *Washington Post*, October 13, 2022.

19. "Two Decades of Change in Federal and State Higher Education Funding," Pew Research Fund, October 15, 2019. See also: Emma Kerr and Sarah Wood, "See the Average College Tuition in 2022–2023," *U.S. News & World Report*, September 12, 2022.

20. Ben Smith, "In 2002 Letter, Paul Wrote of Freedom, Discrimination," *Politico*, May 20, 2010, https://www.politico.com/blogs/ben-smith/2010/05/in-2002-letter-paul-wrote-of-freedom-discrimination-027138.

21. Abby Rapoport, "SREC Member: 'I Got Into Politics to Put Christian Conservatives into Office,'" *Texas Observer*, December 3. 2010.

22. Chris Kromm, "Tea Party Leader: Denying Vote to Those Without Property 'Makes a Lot of Sense,'" *Huffington Post*, December 1, 2010.

23. "No Pay, No Spray: Firefighters Let Home Burn," *NBC News*, October 5, 2010, https://www.nbcnews.com/id/wbna39516346.

24. "Why Firemen Let That House Burn," editorial, *New York Times*, October 6, 2010. See also: "Transcript of the Tuesday Show," *NBC News*, October 5, 2010, https://www.nbcnews.com/id/wbna39536373.

25. "Why Firemen Let That House Burn"; and "Transcript of the Tuesday Show." See also: Armstrong Williams, "Who Is to Blame?" *The Hill*, October 15, 2010.

26. Keith Olberman, "Transcript of the Tuesday Show," *NBC News*, October 5, 2010.

27. Daniel Foster, "Pay-to-Spray Firefighters Watch as Home Burns," *National Review*, October 4, 2010.

28. Bill Press, "Burning Question for the Tea Partyers," *Newsday*, October 10, 2010.

29. Richard Kluger, *Simple Justice: The History of* Brown v. Board of Education *and Black America's Struggle for Equality* (New York: Vintage, 2004), 11–25.

30. Timothy Williams, "Jailed for Switching Her Daughters' School District," *New York Times*, September 26, 2011; see also: "Story of Mother Sentenced to Jail for Enrolling Child in Different District Resurfaced Amid College Scandal," *The Hill*, March 14, 2019; and Annie Lowry, "Her Only Crime Was Helping Her Kids," *The Atlantic*, September 13, 2019; and also "Where School Boundary-Hopping Can Mean Time in Jail," Al Jazeera America, January 21, 2014.

31. Mona Hanna-Attisha, *What the Eyes Don't See: A Story of Crisis, Resistance and Hope in an American City* (New York: One World, 2018).

4. Prophylaxis

1. Mia Ives-Rublee, "As the US Reaches 1 Million Deaths, Congress Still Has Work Ahead," *The Hill*, April 5, 2022.

2. Dean Lueck and Jonathan Yoder, "Spreading like Wildfire," *Regulation*, Health & Medicine, Cato Institute, Winter 2020–2021, pp. 36–42.

3. Dareh Gregorian, "Moderna CEO Grilled over Plan to Raise Covid Vaccine Price at Senate Hearing," *NBC News*, March 22, 2023.

4. "COVID-19 Vaccinations in the United States," Centers for Disease Control, Covid Data Tracker, https://covid.cdc.gov/covid-data-tracker/#vaccinations_vacc-people-booster-percent-pop5.

5. Ethan Cohen and Naomi Thomas, "FDA Vaccine Advisers 'Disappointed' and 'Angry' That Early Data About New Covid-19 Booster Shot Wasn't Presented for Review Last Year," CNN, January 11, 2023.

6. Alex Samuels, "Dan Patrick Says 'There Are More Important Things Than Living and That's Saving This Country,'" *Texas Tribune*, April 20, 2020.

7. *Buckley v. Valeo*, 424 U.S. 1 (1976).

8. *Citizens United v. Federal Elections Commission*, 558 U.S. 310 (2010).

9. *Commonwealth of Massachusetts v. Purdue Pharma*, Superior Court C.A. No. 1884-cv-01808 (BLS2), January 31, 2019.

10. Felix Cohen, "Transcendental Nonsense and the Functional Approach," *Columbia Law Review* 35, no. 6 (June 1935): 809–49.

11. Cohen, "Transcendental Nonsense."

12. Barbara Johnson, "Anthropomorphism in Lyric and Law," *Yale Journal of Law and Humanities* 10 (1998): 549–74, at 549.

13. Annie Karni, "Pence Tours Mayo Clinic and Flouts Its Rule That All Visitors Wear a Mask," *New York Times*, April 28, 2020.

14. Benjamin Swasey, "Pence: 'I Should Have Worn a Mask' When Visiting Mayo Clinic," NPR, May 30, 2020.

15. Swasey, "Pence: 'I Should Have Worn a Mask.'"

16. Keeanga Yamahtta-Taylor, "The Black Plague," *New Yorker*, April 16, 2020.

17. Chinese Exclusion Act of May 6, 1882, Public Law 47-126, Stat. 58, Chap. 126, National Archives.

18. Priscilla Wald, *Contagious: Cultures, Carriers, and the Outbreak Narrative* (Durham, NC: Duke University Press, 2007).

19. Wald, *Contagious*.

20. "NYC Health Department to Spray Pesticides in Certain Neighborhoods," *ABC Eyewitness News*, August 16, 2016. See also: Hannah Frishberg, "Eleven Brooklyn Zip Codes to Be Sprayed for Zika and West Nile Viruses Tonight," *Bklyner*, September 21, 2016.

21. "The Great Barrington Declaration," Open Letter of the American Institute for Economic Research, October 5, 2020. See, in contrast, "The John Snow Memorandum," published in N. A. Alwan et al., "Scientific Consensus on the COVID-19 Pandemic: We Need to Act Now," *The Lancet* 396, no 10260 (October 15, 2020), at e71–e72.

22. Laura Donnely, "Scientists Argue Against Lockdown," *The Telegraph*, October 6, 2020.

23. Sharon Kirkey, "New Declaration Calls for 'Focused Protection' to Achieve COVID-19 Herd Immunity. Critics Say It Would Be Deadly," *National Post*, Toronto, Canada. October 8, 2020.

24. "The Great Barrington Declaration," Open Letter of the American Institute for Economic Research, October 5, 2020.

25. According to the World Health Organization, "'Herd immunity,' also known as 'population immunity,' is the indirect protection from an infectious disease that happens when a population is immune either through vaccination or immunity developed through previous infection. WHO supports achieving 'herd immunity' through vaccination, not by allowing a disease to spread through any segment of the population, as this would result in unnecessary cases and deaths." See: "Herd Immunity, Lockdowns and COVID-19," World Health Organization Report, December 31, 2020.

26. "Herd Immunity," WHO.

27. Bruce Y. Lee, "Trump Says with 'A Herd Mentality' Covid-19 Coronavirus Will Go Away," *Forbes*, September 16, 2020.

28. Killian Meara, "Young Adults with COVID-19 May Have Long-Term Impacts on Blood Vessels, Heart Health," *Contagion Live*, May 13, 2021.

29. "Herd Immunity Letter Signed by Fake Experts Including 'Dr Johnny Bananas,'" *The Guardian*, October 9, 2020. See also: "Dr. Johnny Bananas and Dr. Person Fakename Among Medical Signatories on Herd Immunity Open Letter," *Sky News*, October 9, 2020.

30. John Tamny, "Imagine If the Virus Had Never Been Detected," American Institute for Economic Research, February 4, 2020.

31. Christopher Troeger, "Just How Do Deaths Due to COVID-19 Stack Up?" *Think Global Health*, February 15, 2023.

32. Troeger, "Just How Do Deaths . . . ?"

33. Troeger, "Just How Do Deaths . . . ?"

34. Op-ed, "Biden's Premature Declaration on the End of the COVID-19 Pandemic," *Harvard School of Public Health*, September 27, 2022.

5. Utopia

1. Julie Murphree, "Why in God's Name Are We Growing Cotton in the Desert?" *Arizona Farm Bureau*, May 18, 2016.

2. "Essential Work: Employment and Outlook in Occupations That Protect and Provide," U.S. Bureau of Labor Statistics, September 2020.

3. "Covid-19: Essential Workers in the States," National Conference of State Legislatures, January 11, 2021; and "Executive Order on Protecting Worker Health and Safety," White House, January 21, 2021.

4. United States Flag Code, Title 4, United States Code, Chapter 1, Section 8(j).

5. Upton Sinclair, *The Jungle* (New York: Doubleday, Page, 1906).

6. "The Food and Drug Administration: The Continued History of Drug Advertising," Weill Cornell Medicine, Samuel J. Wood Library and C. V. Starr Biomedical Information Center, New York.

7. Latoya Hill and Samantha Artiga, "COVID-19 Cases and Deaths by Race/Ethnicity: Current Data and Changes over Time," Kaiser Family Foundation, August 22, 2022.

8. Arathi Prasad, "Uché Blackstock: Dismantling Structural Racism in Health Care," *The Lancet* 396, no. 10252 (September 5–11, 2020): 659. See also: Elisabeth Buchwald, "Dispatches from a Pandemic," *Marketwatch*, July 1, 2020.

9. Michael Grabell, "The Plot to Keep Meatpacking Plants Open During COVID-19," *ProPublica*, May 13, 2022.

10. "Families First Coronavirus Response Act: Employee Paid Leave Rights," Wage and Hour Division, U.S. Department of Labor, 2020.

11. Joe Yerardi and Alexia Campbell, "Fewer Inspectors, More Deaths: The Trump Administration Rolls Back Workplace Safety Inspections," *Vox*, August 18, 2020.

6. Making Nice

1. Amy Stamm, "'One Small Step for Man' or 'a Man'?" National Air and Space Museum, *The Smithsonian*, July 17, 2019.

2. "William Shatner Emotionally Describes Spaceflight to Jeff Bezos After Blue Origin Space Launch," *CNBC News*, October 13, 2021.

3. *District of Columbia v. Heller*, 554 U.S. 570 (2008).

4. Neil Vigdor, "Armed Man Who Caused Panic at Missouri Walmart Said It Was 2nd Amendment Test, Authorities Say," *New York Times*, August 9, 2019.

5. Richard Fausset, "A Heavily Armed Man Caused Panic at a Supermarket. But Did He Break the Law?" *New York Times*, January 2, 2023.

6. Zeeshan Aleem, "Lauren Boebert's and Thomas Massie's Christmas Cards Are Disturbing," *MSNBC News*, December 9, 2021.

7. Caroline Light, *Stand Your Ground: A History of America's Love Affair with Lethal Self-Defense* (Boston: Beacon Press, 2018).

8. Fred Barbash, "Florida Police Department Caught Using African American Mug Shots for Target Practice," *Washington Post*, January 16, 2015.

9. The 2022 Florida Statutes, "Justifiable Use of Deadly Force," Title XLVI, Chapter 776, Sect. 776.012, subsect. (1) and (2), l.

10. Tracy Connor, "Florida Deputy Indicted for Killing Jermaine McBean," *NBC News*, December 11, 2015.

11. Kelly Drane, "Every Incident of Mishandled Guns in Schools," Giffords Law Center to Prevent Gun Violence, April 7, 2023.

12. Drane, "Every Incident."

13. Joel Gunter, "After Another Deadly Shooting, Is It Time for Teachers to Carry Guns?" *BBC News*, February 15, 2018. See also: Sarah Mervosh, "Trained, Armed and Ready to Teach Kindergarten," *New York Times*, July 31, 2022.

14. Gunter, "After Another Deadly Shooting."

15. "Gun Suicide Across the States," Fact Sheet, Brady Campaign to Prevent Gun Violence, 2023. See also: David Studdert et al., "Handgun Ownership and Suicide in California," *New England Journal of Medicine* 382, no. 23 (June 4, 2020): 2220–29.

16. "Las Vegas Attack Is Deadliest in Modern US History," Associated Press, October 2, 2017.

17. Mona Chalabi, "How Bad Is US Gun Violence?" *The Guardian*, October 5, 2017.

18. "Firearm Deaths Grow, Disparities Widen," Vital Signs, Centers for Disease Control, 2022.

19. Roberto Esposito, *Persons and Things: From the Body's Point of View* (New York: Polity Press, 2015).

7. Erasure

1. Claudia Schmuckli, ed., *Kehinde Wiley: An Archeology of Silence* (New York: Distributed Art Publishers, 2023).

2. Margaret Burnham, *By Hands Now Known: Jim Crow's Legal Executioners* (New York: Norton, 2023).

3. Burnham, *By Hands Now Known*, xv.

4. *United States v. Cruikshank*, 92 U.S. 542 (1876).

5. Burnham, *By Hands Now Known*, 170.

6. *Screws v. United States*, 325 U.S. 91 (1945).

7. Burnham, *By Hands Now Known*, 173.

8. Burnham, *By Hands Now Known*, 175.

9. Burnham, *By Hands Now Known*, xvi.

10. Burnham, *By Hands Now Known*, xiii.

11. Burnham, *By Hands Now Known*, xvi.

12. Isabel Wilkerson, *The Warmth of Other Suns: The Epic Story of America's Great Migration* (New York: Random House, 2011).

13. Burnham, *By Hands Now Known*, 231.

14. Michael Taussig, *Defacement: Public Secrecy and the Labor of the Negative* (Redwood City, CA: Stanford University Press, 1999).

15. Toni Morrison, "Peril," in *Burn This Book: Notes on Literature and Engagement* (New York: Harper, 2012), 3–4.

16. Margaret Burnham, *By Hands Now Known: Jim Crow's Legal Executioners* (New York: Norton, 2023), 267.

17. "Life Story: Ida B. Wells-Barnett (1862–1931)," from *Black Citizenship in the Age of Jim Crow*, New-York Historical Society, 2022.

18. Photo, Professor Derrick Bell, circa 1990.

19. Hannah Natanson, "It Started with a Mock 'Slave Trade' and a School Resolution Against Racism: Now a War over Critical Race Theory Is Tearing This Small Town Apart," *Washington Post*, July 23, 2021.

20. Natanson, "It Started with a Mock 'Slave Trade.'"
21. Natanson, "It Started with a Mock 'Slave Trade.'"
22. "Draft Diversity, Equity, Belonging and Inclusion Resolution," Travis City Area Public Schools Board of Education, May 21, 2021.
23. Natanson, "It Started with a Mock 'Slave Trade.'"
24. Nikole Hannah-Jones, *The 1619 Project: A New Origin Story* (London: One World, 2021); and Ta-Nehisi Coates, *Between the World and Me* (New York: Spiegel & Grau, 2015).
25. Matthew Schwartz, "Trump Tells Agencies to End Trainings on 'White Privilege' And 'Critical Race Theory,'" *News*, WFDD, Winston-Salem, NC, September 5, 2020.
26. Benjamin Wallace-Wells, "How a Conservative Activist Invented the Conflict over Critical Race Theory, *New Yorker*, June 18, 2021.
27. Wallace-Wells, "How a Conservative Activist Invented the Conflict."
28. Bess Levin, "Trump Tells Supporters They Must Fight to the Death to Stop Schools from Teaching Kids About Systemic Racism," *Vanity Fair*, March 14, 2022.
29. Joseph Goebbels, "The Tasks of the Ministry of Propaganda," speech given to member of the press, March 15, 1933, reprinted in *The Third Reich Sourcebook*, ed. Anson Rabinbach and Sander L. Gilman, trans. Lilian M. Friedberg (Berkeley: University of California Press, 2013).
30. Dennis Romero, "California Man Who Vowed to Bomb Merriam-Webster over Gender-Inclusive Entries Pleads Guilty," NBC News, September 16, 2022.
31. "Update on Book Bans in the 2022–2023 School Year," PEN America Index of School Book Bans. Some of those titles include: Toni Morrison's *Beloved*; Michelle Alexander's *The New Jim Crow*; *The Diary of Ann Frank*; Amnesty International's *We Are All Born Free: The Universal Declaration of Human Rights in Pictures*; Margaret Atwood's *The Handmaid's Tale*; J. M. Barrie's *Peter Pan*; Dinah Brown's *Who Is Malala Yousafzai?*; James Buckley Jr.'s *Who Was Jessie Owens?*; Eric Carle's *Draw Me a Star*; Chief Seattle's *Brother Eagle, Sister Sky*; Cynthia Chin-Lee's *Amelia to Zora: Twenty-Six Women Who Changed the World*; Ta-Nehisi Coates's *Between the World and Me*; Robert Coles's *The Story of Ruby Bridges*; Kathleen Connors's *The Life of Rosa Parks*; Taye Diggs's *Mixed Me!*; Roberta Edwards's *Who Is Barack Obama?*; Sarah Fabiny's *Who Was Frida Kahlo?*; Sarah Fabiny's *Who Was Rachel Carson?*; Jonathan Safran Foer's *Extremely Loud and Incredibly Close*; Jeffrey Fuerst's *African American Cowboys: True Heroes of the Old West*; Catherine Gourley's *Who Was Maria Tallchief?*; Lorraine Hansberry's *A Raisin in the Sun*; James Haskins's *The Scottsboro Boys*; Gail Hernandez's *Who*

Is Derek Jeter?; LeBron James's *I Promise*; Varian Johnson's *What Were the Negro Leagues?*, Katherine Krull's *Starstruck: The Cosmic Journey of Neil deGrasse Tyson*; Harper Lee's *To Kill a Mockingbird*; Grace Lin's *A Big Mooncake for Little Star*; Kevin Noble Maillard's *Fry Bread: A Native American Family Story*; Wynton Marsalis's *Squeak, Rumble, Whomp! Whomp!: A Sonic Adventure*; Nico Medina's *Who Was Aretha Franklin?*; Brad Meltzer's *I Am Martin Luther King, Jr.*; Lupita Nyong'o's *Sulwe*; Andrea Davis Pinkney's *Duke Ellington: The Piano Prince and His Orchestra*; Pam Pollack's *Who Was Lucille Ball?*; Claudia Rankine's *Citizen: An American Lyric*; Dana Meachen Rau's *Who Was Cesar Chavez?*; Arundhati Roy's *The God of Small Things*; Katheryn Russell-Brown's *Little Melba and Her Big Trombone*; Marjane Satrapi's *Persepolis: The Story of a Childhood*; Margot Lee Shetterly's *Hidden Figures: The True Story of Four Black Women and the Space Race*; Sonia Sotomayor's *¡Solo Pregunta!: Se Diferente, Se Valiente, Se Tu* ("Just Ask!: Be Different, Be Brave, Be You"); Art Spiegelman's *Maus*; John Steinbeck's *Of Mice and Men*; William Styron's *The Confessions of Nat Turner*; Susan Verde's *I Am Human: A Book of Empathy*; Kurt Vonnegut's *Slaughterhouse Five*; Mary Dodson Wade's *Condoleeza Rice: Being the Best*; Laurie Wallmark's *Ada Byron Lovelace and the Thinking Machine*; Elie Wiesel's *Night*; Isabel Wilkerson's *Caste: The Origins of Our Discontent*; and August Wilson's play *Fences*. This list is my own culling of PEN's Index, exemplifying to me some of the more troubling eliminations of racial and colonial histories, not to mention PEN's full list of banned material includes hundreds more books having to do with gender, sexuality, women's issues, trans issues, or LGBTQ identities.

8. Process of Elimination

1. Claudia Rupcich, Irina Gonzalez, and Becky Murray, "Toni Morrison's 'Beloved' and 100 Other Books Now Have Warning Labels in Dozens of Florida Schools," *The Skimm*, August 12, 2022, www.theskimm.com/parenting/florida-school-district-books-warning-label.

2. Nathalie Baptiste, "Outrage Over a Single Book Is Shutting Down This Town's Library," AOL, https://www.aol.com/news/outrage-over-single-book-shutting-104500624.html.

3. Matt deGrood, "Huntsville to Pay Private Company to Run City Library Months After Removing LGBTQ+ Display," *Houston Chronicle*, December 21, 2022.

4. Sarah Mervosh, "Florida Scoured Math Textbooks for 'Prohibited Topics.' Next Up: Social Studies," *New York Times*, March 16, 2023.

5. Sarah Mervosh, "Florida Re-edits Another School Subject: Social Studies," *New York Times*, March 17, 2023, p. 1.

6. Mervosh, "Florida Re-edits Another School Subject."

7. Mervosh, "Florida Re-edits Another School Subject."

8. Emma Bowman, "Scholastic Wanted to License Her Children's Book—If She Cut a Part About 'Racism,'" *New York Times*, April 15, 2023.

9. Bowman, "Scholastic Wanted to License Her Children's Book."

10. See the documentary *Coded Bias*, Independent Lens, 2020, available on Netflix.com.

11. Lauren F. Klein, Jacob Eisenstein, and Iris Sun, "Exploratory Thematic Analysis for Digitized Archival Collections," *Digital Scholarship in the Humanities* 30, supplement 1 (December 2015) 130–41.

12. Amardeep Singh, "'Jazz': Map and Quantitative Data," Toni Morrison: A Teaching and Learning Resource Collection, Lehigh University Humanities Lab, 2021, https://scalar.lehigh.edu/toni-morrison/jazz-map-and-quantitative-data?path=maps-and-data.

13. Toni Morrison, *The Source of Self-Regard: Selected Essays, Speeches, and Meditations* (New York: Vintage, 2020).

14. Alex Horton, "Channeling 'The Social Network,' Lawmaker Grills Zuckerberg on His Notorious Beginnings," *Washington Post*, April 11, 2018.

15. Shaila Dewan and Sheera Frenkel, "A Mother, a Daughter, and an Unusual Abortion Prosecution in Nebraska," *New York Times*, August 18, 2022.

16. David Connett, "Women in Finland Post Party Videos to Back PM Sanna Marin," *The Guardian*, August 20, 2022

17. Connett, "Women in Finland Post Party Videos."

18. Anneta Kostantinides, "He Just Wanted to Cuddle! Giant Rat Climbs up Leg and Neck of Sleeping New York Subway Rider," *Daily Mail*, March 29, 2016.

19. Sasha Goldstein, "SEE IT: Huge Rat Climbs Sleeping Man's Neck on 7 Train in Manhattan," *New York Daily News*, March 29, 2016.

20. Ben Feuerherd, "Watch: Rat Crawls up Sleeping Subway Rider's Neck," Channel 4 NBC NewYork News, March 29, 2016.

9. Roots

1. Angela Giuffrida, "'It Is a War': Senator and Auschwitz Survivor Liliana Segre on Fighting Italy's Far Right," *The Guardian*, December 28, 2022.

2. Sherry Turkle, *Reclaiming Conversation: The Power of Talk in a Digital Age* (New York: Penguin Press, 2015).

3. Elaine Scarry, *Thinking in an Emergency* (New York: Norton, 2012).

4. Virginia Eubanks, *Automated Inequality: How High-Tech Tools Profile, Police and Punish the Poor* (London: Picador, 2019).

5. Eubanks, *Automated Inequality*.

6. "Hot Cheeto Girl," entry by "kindagroovin," Urban Dictionary, February 26, 2020.

7. Saidiya Hartman, *Lose Your Mother: A Journey Along the Atlantic Slave Route* (New York: Farrar, Straus and Giroux, 2007).

8. Latoya Hill, Samantha Artiga, and Usha Ranji, "Racial Disparities in Maternal and Infant Health: Current Status and Efforts to Address Them," Kaiser Family Foundation, November 1, 2022.

9. The Butler Act, Tennessee Virtual Archive: Public Acts of the State of Tennessee Passed by the Sixty-Fourth General Assembly, Chapter 27, House Bill No. 185, 1925.

10. Clarence Darrow, *The World's Most Famous Court Trial, State of Tennessee v. John Thomas Scopes: Tennessee Evolution Case*—A Complete Stenographic Report of the Court Test of the Tennessee Anti-Evolution Act, at Dayton, July 10 to 21, 1925, Including Speeches and Arguments of Attorneys (Cincinnati: National Book Co.; New York: Da Capo Press, 1971).

11. Susan Schweik, *The Ugly Laws: Disability in Public* (New York University Press, 2009).

10. Proxy Wars

1. "The Color of Coronavirus: COVID-19 Deaths by Race and Ethnicity in the U.S.," APM Research Lab, April 19, 2023.

2. "The Color of Coronavirus."

3. Tori L. Cowger et al., "Comparison of Weighted and Unweighted Population Data to Assess Inequities in Coronavirus Disease 2019 Deaths by Race/Ethnicity Reported by the US Centers for Disease Control and Prevention," National Library of Medicine, July 1, 2020, *JAMA Network Open* 3, no. 7 (July 2020): e2016933.

4. "Calculators," Medscape, https://reference.medscape.com/guide/medical-calculators.

5. "Fracture Risk Assessment Tool," FRAX calculator at https://frax.shef.ac.uk/FRAX/tool.aspx?country=8. It is worth noting that Country=8 is US (Black), while Country=9 is US (Caucasian).

6. Dorothy Roberts, *Fatal Invention: How Science, Politics and Big Business Recreate Race in the Twenty-First Century* (New York: The New Press, 2012). See also: Jonathan Kahn, *Race in a Bottle: The Story of Bidil and Racialized Medicine in a Post-Genomic World* (New York: Columbia University Press, 2012).

7. Darshali Vyas, Leo Eisenstein, and David Jones, "Hidden in Plain Sight: Reconsidering the Use of Race Correction in Clinical Algorithms," *New England Journal of Medicine* 383, no. 9 (August 27, 2020): 874–82.

8. Lisa Rosenbaum, "Examining Inequity," interview with Marcella Alsan, *New England Journal of Medicine* 388, no. 15 (April 13, 2023): e51.

9. Ariana Eunjung Cha, "Quadriplegic Man's Death from Covid-19 Spotlights Questions of Disability, Race and Family," *Washington Post*, July 5, 2007.

10. Ezekiel J. Emanuel et al., "Fair Allocation of Scarce Medical Resources in the Time of Covid-19," *New England Journal of Medicine* 382, no. 21 (March 23, 2020): 2049–55.

11. Shapiro, 2020.

12. Ari Ne'eman, "I Will Not Apologize for My Needs," *New York Times*, March 23, 2020.

13. Neil Romano, "NCD Chairman Statement on Death of Michael Hickson," National Council on Disability, July 2, 2020.

14. Press Release, "Advocacy Groups and Five Individuals File Discrimination Complaint over COVID-19 Treatment Rationing Guidelines in North Central Texas: Federal Complaint Says North Texas Rationing of Care Guidelines Leave People with Disabilities at Grave Risk," Disability Rights Texas, July 22, 2020.

15. Henry Louis Gates, "My Yiddishe Mama," *Wall Street Journal*, February 1, 2006.

16. Jessie Allen, "A Theory of Adjudication: Law as Magic," *Suffolk University Law Review* 41, no. 4 (2008): 773–831.

17. Blog post, "Is the 'Ashley Treatment' Ethical?" Institute of Clinical Bioethics, Saint Joseph's University, May 1, 2013.

18. Pillowangel.org.

19. Peter Singer, "Opinion: A Convenient Truth," *New York Times*, January 26, 2007.

20. Harriet Washington, *Medical Apartheid: The Dark History of Medical Experimentation on Black Americans from Colonial Times to the Present* (New York: Doubleday, 2007; Anchor, 2008).

21. "The Ashley Treatment: 'Her Life Is as Good as We Can Possibly Make It,'" *The Guardian*, March 15, 2012.

22. Robert Jay Lifton, *The Nazi Doctors: Medical Killing and the Psychology of Genocide* (New York: Basic Books, 1986), 499.

23. Lifton, *Nazi Doctors*, 419.

24. Manny Fernandez and Erik Eckholm, "Pregnant and Forced to Stay on Life Support," *New York Times*, January 7, 2014. See also: Michele Goodwin, *Policing the Womb: Invisible Women and the Criminalization of Motherhood* (Cambridge University Press, 2022).

25. Nikolas Rose, *The Politics of Life Itself: Biomedicine, Power, and Subjectivity in the Twenty-First Century* (Princeton University Press, 2007).

26. Alicia Ouelette, "Eyes Wide Open: Surgery to Westernize the Eyes of an Asian Child," *Hastings Center Report* 39, no. 1 (January–February 2009).

27. Svetlana Boym, *The Future of Nostalgia* (New York: Basic Books, 2002), 117.

11. Dogsbody

1. Christine Hauser, "San Francisco Gallery Owner Is Charged After Spraying Homeless Woman," *New York Times*, January 19, 2023.

2. Dion Lim, "Art Gallery Owner Who Hosed Down Homeless Woman Finds It 'Hard to Apologize,'" ABC Eyewitness News, January 11, 2023.

3. Michel Foucault, *The Birth of the Clinic: An Archeology of Medical Perception* (New York: Vintage, 1994), 6.

4. Nikita Stewart, "Federal Report Finds the City's Rise in Homelessness Went Against a National Trend," *New York Times*, Friday, November 20, 2015, p. A25; Annual Homelessness Assessment Report, Department of Housing and Urban Development, November 19, 2015.

5. "New Yorkers in Need: A Look at Poverty Trends in New York State for the Last Decade," Report issued by the Office of Policy and Analysis, State of New York, December 2022.

12. The Dispossessed

1. Timothy LaHaye and Jerry Jenkins, *Left Behind: A Novel of the Earth's Last Days* (Carol Stream, IL: Tyndale House, 1995).

2. William Luther Pierce, *The Turner Diaries* (Charlottesville, VA: National Vanguard Books, 1978).

3. Henry Wadsworth Longfellow, *Evangeline: A Tale of Acadie* (Boston: Ticknor, 1947; London: Henry Vizetelly, 1850).

4. Samuel Huntington, *The Clash of Civilizations and the Remaking of World Order* (New York: Simon & Schuster, 1996).

5. *Juliana v. United States*, Case No. 20220304_docket-615-cv-01517_response-1.pdf, 2021.

6. "New Orleans Three Years After the Storm: The Second Kaiser Post-Katrina Survey, 2008," Kaiser Family Foundation Report, July 31, 2008.

7. United States Census Bureau, https://data.census.gov/profile?g=160XX00US2255000.

8. Pam Fessler, "After Katrina, New Orleans' Public Housing Is a Mix of Pastel and Promises," NPR, *Morning Edition*, August 17, 2015; and Richard A. Webster, "New Orleans Public Housing Remade After Katrina: Is It Working? *New Orleans Times-Picayune*, August 20, 2015 and July 18, 2019.

9. "Lower Ninth Ward Statistical Area," The Data Center, Nonprofit Knowledge Works, May, 2023

13. The Raw and the Half-Cooked

1. Penelope Green, "Lila Fenwick, Who Broke a Barrier at Harvard Law, Dies at 87," *New York Times*, April 13, 2020.

2. Judith Butler, *Frames of War: When Is Life Grievable?* (Brooklyn: Verso, 2009).

3. Lewis Hyde, *A Primer for Forgetting: Getting Past the Past* (New York: Farrar, Straus and Giroux, 2019).

4. Hyde, *Primer for Forgetting*.

5. Hyde, *Primer for Forgetting*, 29.

6. Michel Foucault, *Power/Knowledge: Selected Interviews and Other Writings 1972–1977*, edited and translated by Colin Gordon et al. (New York: Pantheon, 1980), 119.

7. Martha Minow, *When Should Law Forgive?* (New York: Norton, 2019).

8. Hannah Arendt, *The Human Condition* (Chicago: University of Chicago Press, 1958), 237.

9. Hyde, *Primer for Forgetting*, 66.

10. Hyde, *Primer for Forgetting*, 66.
11. Hyde, *Primer for Forgetting*, 13.
12. Hyde, *Primer for Forgetting*, 50.

14. Gathering the Ghosts

1. Eduardo Cadava, *Paper Graveyards* (Cambridge, MA: MIT Press, 2021).
2. Patricia J. Williams, *Open House: On Family, Food, Friends, Piano Lessons and the Search for a Room of My Own* (New York: Farrar, Straus and Giroux, 2004).
3. Patricia J. Williams, *The Alchemy of Race and Rights: Diary of a Law Professor* (Cambridge, MA: Harvard University Press, 1992).

About the Author

Patricia J. Williams is the James L. Dohr Professor of Law Emerita at Columbia Law School and the longtime former Diary of a Mad Law Professor columnist for *The Nation*. She is a MacArthur fellow and the author of six books, including *The Alchemy of Race and Rights* and *Open House*. She is currently University Distinguished Professor of Law and Humanities at Northeastern University in Boston.

Publishing in the Public Interest

Thank you for reading this book published by The New Press; we hope you enjoyed it. New Press books and authors play a crucial role in sparking conversations about the key political and social issues of our day.

We hope that you will stay in touch with us. Here are a few ways to keep up to date with our books, events, and the issues we cover:

- Sign up at www.thenewpress.com/subscribe to receive updates on New Press authors and issues and to be notified about local events
- www.facebook.com/newpressbooks
- www.twitter.com/thenewpress
- www.instagram.com/thenewpress

Please consider buying New Press books not only for yourself, but also for friends and family and to donate to schools, libraries, community centers, prison libraries, and other organizations involved with the issues our authors write about.

The New Press is a 501(c)(3) nonprofit organization; if you wish to support our work with a tax-deductible gift please visit www.thenewpress.com/donate or use the QR code below.

Other Titles of Interest from The New Press

Administrations of Lunacy: Racism and the Haunting of American Psychiatry at the Milledgeville Asylum
Mab Segrest

Allow Me to Retort: A Black Guy's Guide to the Constitution
Elie Mystal

Blackbirds Singing: Inspiring Black Women's Speeches from the Civil War to the Twenty-first Century
Janet Dewart Bell

Blood on the River: A Chronicle of Mutiny and Freedom on the Wild Coast
Marjoleine Kars

Darker Nations: A People's History of the Third World
Vijay Prashad

Dawn of Detroit: A Chronicle of Slavery and Freedom in the City of the Straits
Tiya Miles

Denmark Vesey's Garden: Slavery and Memory in the Cradle of the Confederacy
Ethan J. Kytle and Blain Roberts

*Fatal Invention: How Science, Politics, and Big Business
Re-create Race in the Twenty-first Century*
Dorothy Roberts

*How We Win the Civil War: Securing a Multiracial Democracy
and Ending White Supremacy for Good*
Steve Phillips

Inventing Latinos: A New Story of American Racism
Laura E. Gómez

*Lighting the Fires of Freedom: African American Women
in the Civil Rights Movement*
Edited by Janet Dewart Bell

Memoir of a Race Traitor: Fighting Racism in the American South
Mab Segrest

Mouths of Rain: An Anthology of Black Lesbian Thought
Edited by Briona Simone Jones

New Jim Crow: Mass Incarceration in the Age of Colorblindness
Michelle Alexander

No More Police: A Case for Abolition
Mariame Kaba and Andrea J. Ritchie

A Perilous Path: Talking Race, Inequality, and the Law
Sherrilyn Ifill, Loretta Lynch, Bryan Stevenson,
and Anthony C. Thompson

Race, Rights, and Redemption: The Derrick Bell Lectures on the Law and Critical Race Theory
Edited by Janet Dewart Bell and Vincent M. Southerland

Thick: And Other Essays
Tressie McMillan Cottom

To Poison a Nation: The Murder of Robert Charles and the Rise of Jim Crow Policing in America
Andrew Baker

The Trials of Madame Restell: Nineteenth-Century America's Most Infamous Female Physician and the Campaign to Make Abortion a Crime
Nicholas L. Syrett

Unreasonable: Black Lives, Police Power, and the Fourth Amendment
Devon W. Carbado

Until We Reckon: Violence, Mass Incarceration, and a Road to Repair
Danielle Sered

Usual Cruelty: The Complicity of Lawyers in the Criminal Injustice System
Alec Karakatsanis

Welcome the Wretched: In Defense of the "Criminal Alien"
César Cuauhtémoc García Hernández

When the Smoke Cleared: The 1968 Rebellions and the Unfinished Battle for Civil Rights in the Nation's Capital
Kyla Sommers

Who Would Believe a Prisoner?: Indiana Women's Carceral Institutions, 1848–1920
The Indiana Women's Prison History Project